EFFECTIVE TEST CONSTRUCTION IN THE HEALTH PROFESSIONS

Harriet L. Schneider, R.N., Ed.D.

Professor, Graduate Faculty, School of Nursing, University of Mississippi at the Medical Center, Jackson.

Formerly Coordinator, Department of Test Development, National League for Nursing, New York.

H. and B. Hess Co., Jackson, Mississippi

ISBN 0-916507-00-9

Printed in the United States of America

TO CAROL HESS-HABER, R.N.,Ph.D.

former student, now stepdaughter,

who said before I married her father,

"You see why you have to be nice to students!

You never know what's going to happen!"

AND

MY NEW AND OLD FAMILIES.

FOREWORD

"How can I tell if my students really know enough to be competent?"

"How can I make my tests better?"

"How come there is not much variation in grades between students? Do they all know the same information or are my tests bad?"

"As a new instructor, how can I find out how to make a test?"

Such questions are often asked by faculty. They are legitimate questions that face all concerned educators. The process of evaluating student performance is not just an administrative necessity or an educational tradition but lies at the heart of the teaching-learning process.

The development of good educational tests is a skill. As a skill, it can be learned and this book should be a valuable help in learning and/or refining the components of this skill. Dr. Schneider's experience as a health care professional, test specialist, and faculty member has provided her with the resources to write a book that is practical and readable. The section on developing the test blueprint will help the reader overcome one of the major flaws in test development, inadequate coverage of behaviors to be tested. Often faculty develop tests that do not cover all of the important domains of behavior. The test blueprint covered in the first chapter will help the reader design the test. This information can then be used to guide the writing of test items. The blueprint can also be valuable in checking to make sure that the final version of the test measures the desired behaviors and content.

The sections on writing various types of questions not only provide the basic rules of item writing but also give examples of errors and the solutions for correcting those errors. Most books about testing give only one or two such examples but this book's many examples make it special. If the reader studies these rules and examples, I believe that better tests will result.

This book should be used by faculty as an introduction to the subject of testing as well as a guide for dealing with problems detected by the item analysis procedures described in the last section of the book.

After reading "Effective Test Construction in the Health Professions" I feel that it will become a valuable reference for faculty to use in their quest to develop better tests.

J. Maurice Mahan, Ph.D.
Director of Instructional Development and Evaluation
University of Mississippi Medical Center

ABOUT THE AUTHOR

Dr. Schneider has written and critiqued thousands of test questions for national standardized examinations (achievement and licensure) in the Department of Test Development at the National League for Nursing over a sixteen-year period. She has served as a consultant to many boards of nursing and has conducted workshops under their auspices. In the last 15 years, she has conducted over 100 workshops on test construction and clinical performance evaluation throughout the United States. The workshop participants and audiences have included, in addition to nurses, physicians, dentists, and other health professionals. Her teaching experience of over ten years has included a diploma program, two baccalaureate nursing programs, and currently a master's degree program in nursing.

PREFACE

This book is the result of the requests of participants at the many workshops I've conducted on Test Construction. In the course of the one- or two-day workshops, I've been asked to spend more time discussing item writing other than multiple-choice questions. Time constraints make that almost impossible because such workshops allow barely enough time to deal with the task of writing effective multiple-choice questions. My philosophy had been that if one can write good multiple-choice questions, in all probability one can write other kinds of questions effectively. There are some similarities but there are also some important differences. I have tried to identify those characteristics in this book. I've also been asked to provide samples of the various types of questions as well as more information about tables of specifications or test blueprints.

People have asked what to look for when critiquing test questions. I have included some of the analytical steps to take in accomplishing that task. To further the analytical process, I have taken questions written mostly by participants and have shown both the original version and my revision of the item. In all instances the intended correct answer has been checked by either me or my tremendously cooperative peers in the School of Nursing of the University of Mississippi at the Medical Center. I, however, assume complete responsibility for the printed correct answer.

Although most of the examples and much of the discussion pertain to nursing, this book should be useful to anyone in any setting who needs to develop questions that truly assess knowledge, particularly at the higher cognitive levels. This is especially true for those in the health professions. It may be used by individuals who wish to improve their skills in item writing, as a supplement to my workshop on test construction, or it may be used in conjunction with other resources in courses on evaluation, measurement and test construction. In all of these situations, I hope it will serve its main purpose--to help you to write better test questions.

No attempt has been made to do an exhaustive job of teaching the user the theoretical foundations of psychometric theory. First, the purpose of this book is to provide specific steps to writing better test questions with examples of the various types. Secondly, the theoretical bases of psychometric theory and the like are very well covered in such classic references as Thorndike and Hagen's Measurement and Evaluation in Psychology and Education. Other excellent resources are given in the section on References. I have not included any sources on the use of computers because I feel that is a subject that deserves a book of its own. (One exception pertains more to item writing than computers per se.) Neither have I included any references on written simulations--they are given (along with an example) in my book Evaluation of Nursing Competence.

ACKNOWLEDGMENTS

Many of the questions were written by participants in the workshops I've conducted on test construction, quite a few by faculty in schools of nursing who submitted them for critique, and a few (especially the questions other than multiple choice) by graduate students in my course. To each of those individuals, I say, "Thank you."

I am indeed grateful to my colleagues in the School of Nursing at the University of Mississippi Medical Center in Jackson. They assisted chiefly by allowing me to try out the questions and answers on them and also in many instances to check out the answers, suggest revisions, and a very important factor, attesting to the face validity of the content. Specifically, I want to say, "Many, many thanks for taking the time in your hectic schedules to help!" Faculty members who went "above and beyond" were Dr. Barbara Boss and Dr. Rene Reeb. They did their usual thorough job. Others who helped a great deal were; Mrs. Delores Barlow, Mrs. Dorothy Crow, Miss Pamela Helms, Miss Kay Lewis, Mr. John Lynn, Mrs. Pepi Nelson, and Mrs. Bobbie Ward. I'd like to thank Dr. June Lawrence who shared questions and item analysis data with me as well as an ear when I needed to discuss a point. Thanks, June! I also want to thank one of my graduate students, Mary Ruth Gibbons, who helped with some of the psychiatric questions.

A very special thank you to a very special person/administrator, my boss, the Associate Dean for Graduate Studies, Dr. Willamay Whitner, who did all she could to facilitate my writing this book. To Dean Edrie George, whom I respect as an administrator and adore as a person, thank you for the privilege of working in a true educational environment.

If I've inadvertently omitted some one, forgive me. I offer a blanket thank you to cover that situation.

CONTENTS

SECTION 1: TEST PLANNING AND BLUEPRINTS

COURSE EVALUATION BLUEPRINTS

An approach that I suggest faculty use before a course is implemented and after the objectives have been written is to design a course evaluation blueprint. This method allows the faculty member to answer the question, "How am I going to evaluate the student's achievement of these objectives?" If the objectives have been written with the same question in mind, (as well as many other pointers), then the objectives can probably be categorized into one of the three domains--cognitive, psychomotor, and affective. (Unfortunately, I have not seen many good examples of objectives in the affective domain that can be assessed.) It should be emphasized at this point that the answers to these questions are global rather than specific. All that is being asked is "Am I going to assess or evaluate this objective in a test, in a nursing care study, or must I observe the student doing something?"

Designing such a blueprint will then lead to the development of other measures such as a test blueprint. All of the objectives that are cognitive and are in the paper-and-pencil column on the evaluation blueprint should be manifested in a test blueprint. A very valuable outcome of designing a course evaluation blueprint is that all of the objectives that are checked in the clinical laboratory column should be the basis of a performance evaluation instrument. Too many times I have found a preponderance of cognitive objectives on a performance evaluation tool. Before you retort with "But nurses don't act in the absence of knowledge! Cognition has to be evaluated, too!", let me reassure you that I agree that cognition needs to be assessed. However, it can be evaluated much more efficiently and reliably in the CLASSROOM. Several examples of course evaluation blueprints follow.

EXAMPLE

EVALUATION BLUEPRINT FOR COURSE EVALUATION (N-007)

OBJECTIVES (N-007)	PAPER & PENCIL TESTS	PERFORMANCE EVALUATION	OTHER TOOLS & TECHNIQUES
I	X		Nursing Process Recording (NPR)
II		X	NPR
III	X		NPR
IV		X	Teaching Project
V	X		IPR
VI	X		Group Community Project
VII		X	NPR
VIII	X		Bibliography Cards
IX	X	X	Teaching Project
X	X	X	Peer evaluations
XI	X	X	Self-evaluation
XII	X	X	Self-evaluation and teacher evaluations

N 4670 CRITICAL CARE NURSING

PORTION OF A COURSE EVALUATION

BLUEPRINT

COURSE OBJECTIVES	HOW/WHERE EVALUATED			
	Paper/ Pencil Tests	Nursing Care Plan	Simulated Laboratory	Clinical Laboratory
1. Perform the following procedures according to the established standards: A. Endotracheal, tracheostomy, and nasopharygeal suctioning B. IV's--initiation, on-going care, administration of medications, discontinuing C. Tracheostomy care D. CVP measurement E. CPR			X	X
2. Describe ICU stressors and patient responses to them in the critical care setting.	X			
3. Explain the procedure for emergency triage and the rationale for it.	X			
4. Describe normal anatomy and physiology of the heart, great vessels and coronary arteries.	X			

COURSE OBJECTIVES	HOW/WHERE EVALUATED			
	Paper/ Pencil Tests	Nursing Care Plan	Simulated Laboratory	Clinical Laboratory
5. Correlate the electrocardiogram with electrical conduction in the heart.	X			
6. Recognize basic cardiac arrhythmias (sinus bradycardia, sinus tachycardia, sinus arrhythmia, sinus arrest, premature atrial contractions, atrial flutter, atrial fibrillation, 1st degree A-V block, premature ventricular contractions, ventricular tachycardia, ventricular fibrillation, asystole) and appropriate pharmacological and/or electrical treatment.	X	X		X
7. Outline nursing assessment and diagnostic studies related to the cardiac patient, including central venous pressure, and pulmonary artery pressures.	X	X		X

PLANNING THE TEST AND TEST BLUEPRINTS

When I was a neophyte instructor, armed with one general course in educational measurement, I would go home over the weekend and both write and type my final exam so I could run it off Monday morning. Obviously, the questions were terrible in terms of what I now know about test construction and it was a very skewed test in relation to content. I was guilty of writing questions in the areas I knew and liked best to the neglect of other equally important content areas. In addition, I am sure the questions were at the lowest levels of the cognitive domain since those questions are the easiest to write. In all probability, I had many questions testing symptoms of diseases and many questions assessing factual knowledge and terminology. I am not negating the fact that these areas should be tested but rather that there should have been more questions assessing application and analysis. Another way of making my point is to say I should have asked more questions aimed at applying those facts. For example, because a patient has a low white blood cell count, what does the nurse need to know or do or prevent or watch for?

An approach that is advocated to avoid constructing a test that is skewed both in content and in cognitive levels is to construct a table of specifications or test blueprint or test grid. By putting down in black and white what a particular test will cover will help to systematically sample from the universe of content for that specific subject. In addition, if cognitive levels are also included, it may help to ensure that more than facts and terminology are included. A word of caution, however. It is neither easy to write questions at a given higher cognitive level nor guaranteed that questions for individual students will assess that particular cognitive level. For example, what may be application for one student may be simply recall for another student, depending on the student's experiences. It is well to remember that to test for application of knowledge, one must present the student with a new or novel situation. If one simply asks what was presented directly in class or "lifts" statements from textbooks, what is tested is usually recall.

But to get back to the test blueprint. There are a variety of ways to approach the development of a table of specifications. One can use objectives, broad content areas, cognitive levels, actual ideas for test questions in each of the cells of the grid, numbers of items in each of the cells and/or percentages of items, or any combination of the above. I personally prefer to include both actual ideas for questions and the number of items to be included. It is easier, I believe, to fill in the cells in relation to ideas for questions as one is preparing material for the classes that correspond with that area. In addition, it is probably easiest to actually write the questions at that point because the content is fresh in one's head. Also, since I advocate validating the correct answer along with the item, it will be easiest and less time-consuming to do so at the same time.

Many of the objectives an instructor creates for a course, unit, or class are measurable by paper-and-pencil tests. These objectives may be listed along one dimension of a test grid while the other dimension may be related to content (subject matter), ages and/or stages of development, complexity of care required by clients, locus of decision making, levels of wellness, body systems and on and on. My point here is that questions can be written to assess student's achievement of those objectives. Most of the time, a number of questions can be written for each objective. If the questions are coded and filed appropriately, they can be retrieved whenever it is necessary to put together a test. By building up a reservoir of test questions, it theoretically is possible to put together a new test every time. I am highly in favor of this practice because I have seen what happens when old copies of exams are made available to students. They can memorize that content but that's all!

I am sure you will agree with me that we must prepare students to function in the real world at a level of competence above the ability to recite facts! More and more we are hearing about the need to prepare practitioners to function in this highly technological society with our current knowledge having a very short life. We need to prepare students to make judgements, problem-solve, be creative in the solution to old and new problems, and to be leaders in their chosen professions.

Our test questions can reflect those high level objectives and students' responses to those questions can be very informative about where they are in relation to meeting those objectives. We are at the same time conveying to the students that we expect more of them than simple recall and memorization of facts.

Included in the section on multiple-choice questions are a number of objectives and test items written to those objectives. They illustrate how test questions can be structured to help assess achievement of those objectives.

Several examples of test blueprints follow and in some instances, only a part of a blueprint is shown. Let me emphasize that there are a variety of approaches to developing a test grid and the one you design should meet your needs. For further information on the use of tables of specifications, consult any of the good psychometric references. I have also included my version of a portion of a test blueprint for the new licensing examination for registered nurses. (I hope you note that regardless of the format of the blueprint, important content is important content and should be reflected in the blueprint.)

SAMPLE OF A TEST BLUEPRINT
FOR A NURSING OF CHILDREN EXAMINATION

COGNITIVE LEVELS / AGES	NUMBER OF ITEMS BY AGE GROUPS									TOTAL
	Infancy 22		Preschool years 22		Early school years 22		Adolescence 10		General 24	100
1. Knowledge of terms	normal	1	normal	1	normal	1	normal	1	2	8
	sick	1	sick	0	sick	1	sick	0		
2. Knowledge of facts, principles and methods	normal	3	normal	3	normal	2	normal	1	2	20
	sick	3	sick	3	sick	2	sick	1		
3. Application of facts and principles and evaluation of evidence (other than 4)	normal	3	normal	3	normal	4	normal	2	10	39
	sick	5	sick	5	sick	6	sick	1		
4. Application of psychosocial facts and principles and evaluation of evidence	normal	3	normal	4	normal	3	normal	2	10	33
	sick	3	sick	3	sick	3	sick	2		

TIME: TWO HOURS.

ITEMS: 100 FOUR-OPTION MULTIPLE CHOICE.

PORTION OF A TEST BLUEPRINT REFLECTING MY IMPRESSION OF APPROPRIATE CONTENT FOR THE NATIONAL COUNCIL LICENSURE EXAMINATION FOR REGISTERED NURSES (NCLEX-RN)

CONTENT / BEHAVIORS	ASSESSING	ANALYZING	PLANNING	IMPLEMENTING	EVALUATING
Normal Newborn	Apgar Score @ 1 & 5 minutes	Bilirubin lab results	Spits up formula-- observe mother feed	Care of umbilical cord that is moist	Physical Appraisal
Normal Pregnant Woman	Ankles edematous-- get history re rest and Na intake	Urine contains sugar but no acetone	Follow-up after teaching about nutrition	Teaching her about nutrition, etc.	On return visit, check her for edema

PORTION OF A TEST BLUEPRINT FOR A COURSE
IN GROWTH AND DEVELOPMENT OF THE CHILD

CONTENT / AGES	NEWBORN	INFANT	TODDLER
FEEDING AND NUTRITION	First feedings - breast artificial	Introduction of solid foods Weaning	Self-feeding problems
ELIMINATION	Description of normal stools	Relationship of diet to stools Capacity of bladder	Toilet-training
SLEEPING	Sleep patterns	Sleep patterns	Delay at bed-time Early wake-up problems
IPR AND SOCIALI-ZATION	Specific mother-figure less important	Age of response to mother's voice Fear of strangers	Parallel play Reaction to a new sibling
PHYSICAL DEVELOPMENT	Characteristics of the newborn	Rolling over Pincer-finger skills Sitting up Standing Tooth eruption	Safety re mobility Walking skills Push-pull toys

SECTION 2: WRITING TEST QUESTIONS WITH EXAMPLES OF EACH TYPE

GENERAL GUIDES FOR WRITING TEST QUESTIONS

1. Test only meaningful content, not trivia!
2. Keep the reading level of the question low--you want to test nursing knowledge, not reading comprehension.
3. Textbooks may be used for validating content but direct statements or content should not become the basis of the question. In other words, do not lift sentences from the book since this tests only memory. Additionally, this practice results in testing only facts as compared to the application of such facts.
4. Avoid tricky questions!
5. Be careful to avoid providing clues to other questions. This can occur in the stem of the question, in headings of sections (if they are used), and also in the history or patient situation. It is essential to read over the entire assembled test before it is typed to make sure this has not happened.
6. In general, items should stand alone--be independent of one another. There are exceptions to this maxim such as in written simulation examinations.
7. Try to avoid writing questions that may be interpreted differently by students with varying backgrounds. One pitfall in item writing is the unintentional writing of ambiguous questions. Have a peer read them before they are tried out on students just to be sure that you have communicated your intent.
8. In order to test for the application of knowledge, the student must be presented with a new or novel situation.
9. Include the authority in the stem of the question if the content to be tested is based on that authority.The same practice is true in regard to opinions.
10. Avoid systematic response patterns--they should be random.

COMMON FAULTS IN WRITING MULTIPLE CHOICE QUESTIONS WITH SIX EXAMPLES

In the course of critiquing thousands of test questions written by faculty in different disciplines, I have identified six reoccurring faults in the writing of multiple-choice questions. These 6 faults are;

1. The correct answer is longer and/or more specific than the distractors.
2. The options are constructed in overlapping quantities so that the intended correct answer appears in more than 1 option.
3. A grammatical clue in the stem of the question leads to the correct answer.
4. There is a direct association between the stem of the question and the correct answer.
5. Qualifying words or specific determiners are used in the distractors and not in the correct answer.
6. More than 1 part or point is included in the correct answer while each of the distractors includes only 1 part or point.

The examples that follow illustrate each type of fault. Where underlining has been used, its purpose is to identify the fault(s) in item construction.

NOTE: An asterisk * has been used throughout the text to indicate the correct answer in the multiple-choice questions.

LONGER CORRECT ANSWER

1. When a cough mixture is administered to a patient, it should be
   - A. consumed slowly.
   - B. held in the mouth before swallowing.
   - C. diluted, followed immediately with water.
   - * D. undiluted and the patient instructed not to drink immediately after it has been taken.

OVERLAPPING QUANTITIES

2. The normal range of cerebral spinal fluid pressure is
   - A. 25 - 90 mm H_2O
   - * B. 60 - 180 mm H_2O
   - C. 150 - 250 mm H_2O
   - D. 260 - 380 mm H_2O

NOTE: Both options A and C contain parts of the correct answer. The range varies from option to option, too.

GRAMMATICAL CLUE

3. After an intramuscular needle has been inserted into the tissue, <u>what precaution</u> should the nurse take before injecting the medication?
   1. Decrease the angle of the needle to the skin.
   2. Draw back on the plunger to aspirate fluid.
   3. Lift up the tissue surrounding the injection site.
   4. Check the attachment of the needle to the syringe.

- * A. <u>2 only</u>.
- B. 1 and 3.
- C. 2 and 4.
- D. 1, 2, and 4
- E. All of them.

CLUE IN STEM TO CORRECT ANSWER

4. A patient who will have an incision in the right upper quadrant of his abdomen is taught how to cough postoperatively. Which of the following measures will help to decrease discomfort in the <u>incisional</u> area when he coughs postoperatively?

   A. Turning onto his left side.

   B. Lowering the head of his bed.

   * C. Supporting his <u>incision</u> with a pillow.

   D. Bending his head forward, toward his chest.

SPECIFIC DETERMINERS IN DISTRACTORS

5. A new mother is concerned because her 36-hour-old infant has a purulent discharge from his eyes, and the skin around his eyes is slightly discolored. Which of these actions by the nurse would be best?

   * A. Explaining to the mother that the discharge is probably due to the silver nitrate that was instilled at birth and will gradually disappear.

   B. Telling the mother that the discharge is probably due to a Neisserian infection and that the baby should probably be isolated.

   C. Informing the mother that <u>all</u> newborn babies have this condition.

   D. Giving <u>no</u> information to the mother about her baby's condition.

NOTE: The correct answer and distractor B contain qualities, i.e., <u>probably</u>.

MULTIPLE PARTS IN CORRECT ANSWER

6. The most therapeutic verbal communication occurs when the nurse

   A. guides the interaction by asking questions about the client's problems.

   B. gives advice to the client to help him solve his problems.

   * C. listens to the client and verbally focuses and seeks clarification.

   D. seeks opportunities to enhance the client's self-esteem.

In becoming familiar with these common faults in item writing, it will help you to avoid committing them yourself. In addition, it should be useful to you when critiquing the questions of your peers.

EXAMPLES OF WHAT NOT TO DO!

One of the maxims of item writing is to avoid providing clues to the correct answer. Look at this example:

> It is difficult to obtain valid data when one is a participant observer chiefly because
>
> 1. the method is time-consuming.
> 2. the observer may lose objectivity.
> 3. the behavior will probably be difficult to describe.
> 4. the technique closely resembles interview technique.

The clue word in the stem of the question and in the correct answer (2) is OBSERVER. It is also wise to avoid using clue words in the wrong choices or distractors. If this is done, the test-wise student and some of the less knowledgeable students may select the option that contains the clue. It is not uncommon for students to label such questions "tricky" and I believe they are justified.

It is sound test construction practice to avoid labeling parts of the test with the subject matter or content that will follow. Look at the following example:

> INFLAMMATION
>
> 1. New ostomies should have the bag changed initially every day because of the
>   1. unsightly contents.
>   2. need to eliminate odor.
>   3. shrinkage of the stoma.
>   4. possibility of infection.

In this example, the clue word in the correct answer (4) is infection which is the only choice that pertains to the heading INFLAMMATION. A student just needs to be test wise to get this question correct.

GUIDELINES FOR WRITING MULTIPLE-CHOICE QUESTIONS

1. Write test questions that assess important learning outcomes. Avoid testing trivia!

2. Include only one significant problem in the stem of the question. The stem should be meaningful by itself. You should not have to read all of the choices to make sense out of the question.

3. Use simple, clear language in presenting the complete problem in the stem. Your questions should assess nursing knowledge not reading comprehension.

4. Make sure that the problem in the stem is accurate and reflects current practice--has face validity.

5. Include as much information as possible in the stem of the question. This practice will often help to make the options short and cut down on the amount of reading. There are instances, however, when it is wise to repeat common words in the options for greater clarity or grammatical consistency.

6. Include in the stem of the question only the information needed to answer the question. Extraneous material may make the question more interesting but may also confuse the examinee. However, in certain circumstances you may want to assess students' problem-solving ability to sort out relevant from irrelevant material necessary to solve the problem. In this situation, it will obviously be necessary to include such data.

7. Whenever possible, word the stem of the question in positive form. Using the negative approach necessitates two steps in answering the question--first identifying the "good" or correct options before going on to identify the "bad" or wrong choices.

8. If it is necessary to use negative wording in the stem, capitalize and underscore the negative word or words. However, underlining of other words is generally discouraged. The overuse of underlining negates the purpose and loses its impact.

9. It is easier for students to answer questions if the options come at the end of the stem. Do not leave blank spaces in the middle of the stem.

10. Make sure that there is only one clearly correct or best answer to each question! Authorities in the subject area should agree with the selected choice. Document or validate the correct answer as completely as possible.

11. Make sure that each distractor sounds plausible and will appeal to at least some of the uninformed examinees. If a distractor is not chosen by anyone, it makes no contribution to the item and should be either revised or eliminated. Exceptions to this maxim involve items that are very easy--say 95% to 100% of the students getting the answer right--and items involving mastery of content when hopefully the majority of the students will also get the answer right.

    Before a distractor can be selected by an examinee, it must be familiar to the student. A chemistry test or blood test that doesn't exist or a drug that has been made up by some creative faculty member is a "no-no."

12. Make sure that all options are grammatically correct and that they either complete the stem of the item or "fit" with the completed stem.

13. Try to word options in parallel form whenever possible using comparable grammatical structure.

14. Options that are in logical order make it easier for examinees to respond to the question--to find the correct answer, assuming they know it.

15. Make sure that variations in options involving quantities do not give clues to the correct answer. Keep the amounts as consistent as possible but of course, plausible.

16. The difficulty of test items may often be adjusted by changing options. For example, the same question may be used with practical nurses and registered nurses. What should be different are the sets of options offered to each.

17. To avoid providing unintended clues to the correct answer, make sure there is no consistent pattern either in length or in the complexity of the correct answer. It is well to remember that since the correct answer often needs to be qualified, it tends to be longer than the distractors. Therefore, an effort should be made to avoid this practice.

18. The correct answers in a test should be randomly assigned whenever possible. It should appear in each position approximately an equal number of times. If the options are logically organized or involve numbers, do not randomize those answers.

19. Avoid verbal clues or associations that may be helpful to students in selecting the correct answer and/or in eliminating distractors. This practice involves not only false or irrelevant clues, but also words that sound alike in the stem and options (associations.)

20. In the typical multiple-choice test format, make certain that each item is independent of other items in the test. (Exceptions to this maxim include written simulations and patient management problems.)

21. In the preparation of the total test, make sure that all parts of a question are on the same page. An exception to this maxim might be the inclusion of pictorial material such as a graph, chart, diagram and the like in a separate section or on a separate page.

    Spacing between questions and options should be generous enough to facilitate reading.

22. For combination-type multiple-choice questions, use the options "all of the above" and "none of the above" with caution. Most faculty tend to make "all of the above" the correct answer each time it is used rather than only about 25% of the time.

    When knowing what not to do is important, "none of the above" may be very appropriate. When used in this manner, remember to also use it as an incorrect answer some of the time. It is also important to remember that "none of the above" requires two words in the stem to make that option plausible, namely, "if any."

23. In writing items at the application level, some new or novel aspect needs to be included in the question. If the item contains content that is almost identical to what has been taught in class, the students' responses will be based on memory rather than the application of knowledge.

24. If it is necessary to write an "except" question, the following stem seems to cause the least difficulty for examinees.

    Three of the following symptoms (or whatever) occur early in the development of X. Which one is the <u>EXCEPTION</u>?

INTRODUCTION TO THE EXAMPLES OF MULTIPLE-CHOICE QUESTIONS THAT FOLLOW

I have taken fourteen multiple-choice questions submitted for critique and have revised them according to the guidelines just presented. Each of the questions is on a separate page. Below I have listed the page number and the guidelines that were violated for the item on that page. Other considerations that may have entered into my decision to revise the item may also be offered. Those considerations include; general appearance of the item, consistency in format, mixing lay terminology with medical terminology and the like. Sometimes it was a matter of wording it differently for clarity (stem and/or options), punctuation that was inappropriate, capital letters that should have been lower case ones and vice versa. In all instances, I did have a reason, albeit an unwritten one.

My suggestion to you is to first critique the items according to the guidelines to see if you can identify any problems with them. Then come back to these two pages to check your results with those presented here.

CRITIQUE OF QUESTIONS

Page 25 The stem neither asks a question nor is it an open-ended stem completed by the options. Only 2 parts of the options were repeated--feedback and tension. I added 2 other pairs--conflict and equifinality to hopefully increase their plausibility. I believe the stem is clearer now. Guideline #12 was violated.

Page 26 Guidelines #8, 10, and 17 were violated. The correct answer originally was the only one with 2 parts.

Page 27 Guidelines #5, 8, 12, 13, and 22 were violated.

Page 28 Guidelines #13 and 19 were violated. There is a clue to the correct answer in the stem--Mrs.Smith. I also added quotes to each option.

Page 29 Guidelines #11 and 19 were violated. There is a clue to the correct answer--sugar is in the stem.

Page 30 Guidelines #6, 8, and 19 were violated.

Page 31 Guidelines #6, 13, and 19 were violated.

Page 32 Guideline #6 was violated. There was no question mark in the original.

Page 33 Guidelines #6, 11, and 13 were violated.

Page 34 The original version of this item gave all parts of the options in rows across the page rather than in a list, which are easier to answer. Guidelines #13, 14, and 15 were violated.

Page 35 Guidelines #6, 13, and 14 were violated.

Page 36 Guidelines #9, 13, and 15 were violated.

Page 37 Guidelines #4 and 22 were violated.

Page 38 Guidelines #11 and 13 were violated. The correct answer had 2 parts and the others had only one.

ORIGINAL VERSION

Because social systems are continuously involved in the processes of (select one option from below) they tend to be in a constant state of disorganization or disequilibrium.

1. Input, output and feedback.
2. Stress, conflict and succession.
3. Feedback, tension and homeostasis.
4. Tension, equifinality and prediction.

REVISED VERSION

Social systems tend to be in a constant state of disorganization or disequilibrium because they are continuously involved in the processes of

* 1. input, output, and feedback.
2. stress, conflict, and equifinality.
3. feedback, tension, and homeostasis.
4. tension, equifinality, and conflict.

ORIGINAL VERSION

When giving an intramuscular injection in the mid-anterior thigh, which of the following must be avoided?

1. Sciatic nerve
2. Femoral artery and vein
3. Gluteal artery
4. Inguinal fossa

REVISED VERSION

When giving an intramuscular injection in the mid-anterior thigh (vastus lateralis site), which of the following structures must be AVOIDED?

1. Inguinal fossa
2. Ventrogluteal area
3. * Femoral artery and vein
4. Sciatic notch and nerve

ORIGINAL VERSION

Which of the following is not true regarding brushing the hair?

1. helps keep the hair clean.
2. stimulates the circulation of blood in the scalp.
3. decreases the amount of oil along each hair shaft.
4. prevents accumulative matting and tangling.
5. none of the above.

REVISED VERSION

Which of the following benefits, if any, is INCORRECT in relation to brushing one's hair?

1. It helps to keep the hair clean.
2. It prevents accumulative matting and tangling.
3. It stimulates the circulation of blood in the scalp.
4. * It decreases the amount of oil along each hair shaft.
5. None of them.

ORIGINAL VERSION

Mrs. Smith had major abdominal surgery yesterday. Which approach would be best to make initially in talking with her about taking a bath?

1. How have you been taking your bath?
2. Mrs. Smith, it's time for your bath.
3. Do you need any help with your bath?
4. Time to wake up--it's time for our bath.

REVISED VERSION

Mrs. Smith had major abdominal surgery yesterday. Which of these approaches regarding her morning bath would it be best to make initially?

* 1. "Mrs. Smith, it's time for your bath."
2. "Time to wake up, Mrs. Smith--it's time for our bath."
3. "Do you need any help with your bath, Mrs. Smith?"
4. "How have you been taking your bath, Mrs. Smith?"

ORIGINAL VERSION

If a patient's breakfast tray was marked with a regular diet card and he asked for more sugar for his cereal, you would:

1. Get more sugar for him.
2. Ask the head nurse if he can have more.
3. Try to convince the patient that he doesn't need it.
4. Explain that the correct amount for a regular diet is placed on his tray.

REVISED VERSION

A regular diet is prescribed for a patient and he receives the appropriate breakfast tray. He asks the nurse for additional sugar for his cereal. What would it be best to do?

* 1. Get more sugar for him.
2. Ask the nurse in charge if he may have more sugar.
3. Try to convince the patient that he doesn't really need more sugar.
4. Explain to the patient that the recommended amount for his type of diet was placed on his tray.
5. Offer to get the patient a sugar substitute, while acquainting him with the adverse effects of excessive sugar consumption.

ORIGINAL VERSION

T. Swift, nursing student, will be taking his adult client's rectal temperature shortly. The student realizes that which of the following would not be correct for him to implement:

1. obtain a stubby or blunt bulbed thermometer.
2. omit the use of a lubricant as the rectum secretes one itself.
3. insert the thermometer about 1½ inches.
4. leave the thermometer in place three (3) minutes.

REVISED VERSION

In taking an adult's rectal temperature, 3 of the following steps are correct. Which one is INCORRECT?

* 1. Omitting the use of a lubricant.
2. Obtaining a stubby or blunt bulbed thermometer.
3. Inserting the thermometer about one and a half inches.
4. Leaving the thermometer in place approximately three minutes.

ORIGINAL VERSION

You cannot obtain an ausculatory blood pressure on your client so you know you must take a palpatory. A palpatory B/P is an estimate of the:

1. diastolic blood pressure.
2. systolic and diastolic pressure.
3. pulse pressure.
4. systolic pressure.

REVISED VERSION

A palpatory blood pressure is an estimate of the

1. pulse pressure.
2. diastolic pressure.
* 3. systolic pressure.
4. diastolic and systolic pressure.

ORIGINAL VERSION

N. Nifty, nursing student, is caring for an adult client with a respiratory infection. She is aware that her client will be experiencing pyrexia. Which is the most consistent sign or symptom of pyrexia that she be alert to:

1. dyspnea.
2. diaphoresis.
3. decreased systolic B/P.
4. increased pulse rate.

REVISED VERSION

The most consistent sign or symptom of pyrexia is

1. dyspnea.
2. diaphoresis.
3. * increased pulse rate.
4. decreased systolic blood pressure.

ORIGINAL VERSION

You count Mr. Heart's radial pulse and find it to be irregular. You realize that you must obtain an apical-radial pulse. This is determined by:

1. taking the apical pulse first, then the radial and making a comparison.
2. one nurse taking the apical pulse and another nurse taking the radial pulse at the same time and then making a comparison.
3. two nurses counting the pulse deficit.
4. subtracting the radial pulse from the apical pulse.

REVISED VERSION

An apical-radial pulse is determined by

1. counting the apical pulse first, then counting the radial pulse and subtracting it from the apical pulse.
2. counting the radial pulse first, then counting the apical pulse and subtracting it from the radial pulse.
3. * having one nurse take the apical pulse at the same time that another nurse is taking the radial pulse and then making a comparison.
4. having two nurses each take both the apical and radial pulses and then taking the average of each.

MULTIPLE-CHOICE

Which of the following groups of characteristics can be identified in the EKG strip shown below?

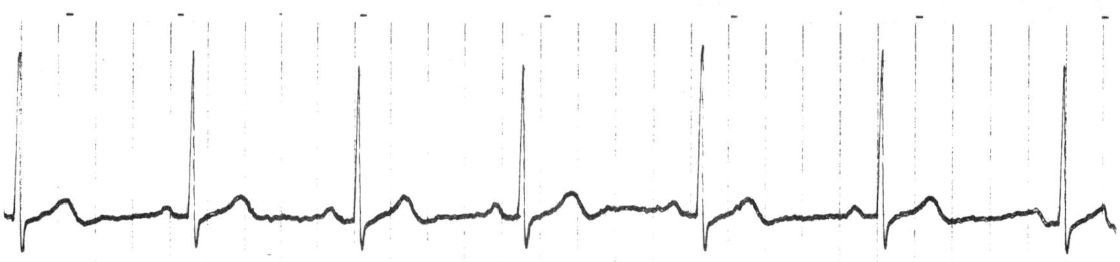

1. Rate - 30
   Rhythm - irregular
   P waves - present
   P-R interval - 0.12 seconds
   QRS - 0.16 seconds

2. Rate - 60
   Rhythm - irregular
   P waves - absent
   P-R interval - 0.40 seconds
   QRS - 0.08 seconds

* 3. Rate - 60
   Rhythm - regular
   P waves - present
   P-R interval - 0.16 seconds
   QRS - 0.06 seconds

4. Rate - 100
   Rhythm - regular
   P waves - absent
   P-R interval - 0.22 seconds
   QRS - 0.10 seconds

ORIGINAL VERSION

Betty, a 10-month-old infant, is seen in the well child clinic at Southern Health Center. The mother states that she has had all her immunizations for her age. Based on the American Academy of Pediatrics, recommendations for beginning age, and immunization schedule, you would know that she has been immunized against

1. whooping cough, diphtheria, scarlet fever, polio
2. diphtheria, polio, tetanus, measles
3. pertussis, polio, measles, tetanus
4. tetanus, pertussis, polio, diphtheria

REVISED VERSION

A 10-month-old infant has received all of her immunizations. According to the recommendations of the American Academy of Pediatrics, this means that this infant has been immunized against

1. diphtheria, scarlet fever, polio, and measles.
2. diphtheria, scarlet fever, tetanus, and measles.
3. tetanus, pertussis, polio, and measles.
* 4. tetanus, pertussis, polio, and diphtheria.

ORIGINAL VERSION

The head is the presenting part in _______ percent of all deliveries.

a. 30%

b. 50%

c. 60%

d. more than 95%

REVISED VERSION

The head is the presenting part in approximately what percent of all deliveries?

A. 30%

B. 50%

C. 75%

* D. 95%

ORIGINAL VERSION

An epidural hematoma is usually a result of:

a. arterial bleeding
b. venous bleeding
c. oozing cerebral spinal fluid
d. none of the above

REVISED VERSION

An epidural or extradural hematoma usually results from which of the following, if any, causes?

A. Arterial bleeding.
B. Venous bleeding.
C. Oozing cerebral spinal fluid.
* D. None of them.

DISCUSSION:

In the original question, the correct answer was not indicated. In checking the literature for the correct answer, I found the following;

"Laceration of the middle meningeal artery and/or vein is the source of the hemorrhage" under a discussion of extradural or epidural hematoma. The reference I used was by Joanne Hickey and titled The Clinical Practice of Neurological and Neurosurgical Nursing. It was published in 1981 by J.B. Lippincott Company in Philadelphia.

Perhaps it would be best to revise the options completely. The correct answer could be worded something like "bleeding from the middle meningeal artery and/or vein."

ORIGINAL VERSION

The overall goal in the treatment of ulcerative colitis is to

1. rest bowel and promote healing.
2. prevent reoccurrence.
3. prevent complications.
4. promote nutrition.

REVISED VERSION

The overall goal in the treatment of clients with ulcerative colitis is to

* 1. rest the bowel and promote healing.
2. prevent complications or its reoccurrence.
3. promote nutrition and decrease the number of stools.
4. restore normal body flora and prevent infection.

While samples of questions illustrating all of the violations of guidelines were not presented, the ones that were demonstrated some of the most common problems. I hope that you were able to identify a good many of those problems. I often have to remind people that item writing is a skill that one develops over time--it is not accomplished instantly! Being aware of the major, common flaws in item writing is the first step to improving your own questions.

INTRODUCTION TO THE MULTIPLE-CHOICE QUESTIONS WRITTEN TO OBJECTIVES

The need to assess the attainment or achievement of educational objectives is frequently heard in academic circles. Among those objectives are the ones in the cognitive domain and these can be assessed effectively by multiple-choice questions (except for the level of synthesis which cannot be assessed in this manner.) Such objectives can be course objectives, unit objectives, or daily objectives. Each objective, regardless of level, can probably be used as the basis for several questions. The more important the objective and the more general the objective, the more test questions that can be written to that objective. The more specific the objective, the more creative the item writer will need to be to write several test questions to assess that objective.

For your own purposes, it is wise to keep a record of which test questions go with which objectives. This can be accomplished quite easily on item analysis cards. Section 4 deals with item analysis and item analysis cards. A word of caution--when your tests are typed and reproduced, do not include the objectives (either written out or just by its number) because it may provide a clue to the correct answer.

In the section that follows, I have provided a variety of objectives with one test question written to each. These objectives and the accompanying questions were written by workshop participants and have been revised by me in keeping with principles of item writing. The correct answers, which most of the time were not provided, have been checked for accuracy.

A MULTIPLE-CHOICE QUESTION TO AN OBJECTIVE

OBJECTIVE:

Identify expansion of the chief complaint as being the first step in obtaining a health history.

QUESTION:

A client complains of being constipated for the past three weeks. Which of the following questions should be asked first?

* 1. "What do you mean by 'constipation'?"
2. "What medications are you now taking?"
3. "Has anyone else in your family been constipated?"
4. "Has there been a change in your diet habits?"

A MULTIPLE-CHOICE QUESTION TO AN OBJECTIVE

OBJECTIVE:

Identify the appropriate medical aseptic practice in the care of patients with type B hepatitis.

QUESTION:

When caring for a patient with type B hepatitis, caution must be exercised with which of the following items?

1. Stool and urine.
* 2. Needle and syringe.
3. Linen and eating utensils.
4. Nasal and oral secretions.

A MULTIPLE-CHOICE QUESTION TO AN OBJECTIVE

OBJECTIVE:

Institutes appropriate nursing intervention to treat a hypoglycemic reaction in an insulin-dependent client.

QUESTION:

Mrs. Kline, 40 years old, has diabetes mellitus. She received 40 units of NPH insulin at 7:30 A.M.

At 4:00 P.M. Mrs. Kline says that she has a headache and she is diaphoretic and irritable. The initial nursing action should be to

1. take all of her vital signs.
2. test her urine for glucose and acetone.
3. give her concentrated carbohydrate. *
4. give her regular insulin coverage as prescribed.

A MULTIPLE-CHOICE QUESTION TO AN OBJECTIVE

OBJECTIVE:

Predict treatment modalities for clients with cancer.

QUESTION:

Which of these treatment modalities is most appropriate for a client who has oat cell cancer of the lung?

1. Interferon therapy.
2. Surgical intervention.
3. * Chemotherapy and radiotherapy.
4. Hyperthermia and oxygen therapy.

A MULTIPLE -CHOICE QUESTION TO AN OBJECTIVE

OBJECTIVE:

Identifies appropriate nursing measures associated with the care of the laboring woman receiving analgesia/anesthesia.

SITUATION:

Mrs. Mary Samet, a 22-year-old primigravida, is in active labor. She has just received an epidural and is on her back with her head slightly elevated. The nurse monitors Mrs. Samet's blood pressure and finds that it has dropped from 120/70 to 110/58 in a 10-minute period. Mrs. Samet says to the nurse, "I feel funny."

The most appropriate action by the nurse would be to

1. assess her cervical dilatation.
2. examine her for vaginal bleeding.
3. place her in Trendelenburg's position.
* 4. turn her onto her left side.

A MULTIPLE-CHOICE QUESTION TO AN OBJECTIVE

OBJECTIVE:

Demonstrates knowledge of the concept of pulse pressure as it relates to cardiac stroke volume.

QUESTION:

Which of the following understandings about pulse pressure as it relates to shock is accurate?

1. An increase in pulse pressure is more significant than is the blood pressure.

* 2. A decrease in pulse pressure is more significant than is the blood pressure.

3. Pulse pressure and blood pressure are equally significant.

A MULTIPLE-CHOICE QUESTION TO AN OBJECTIVE

OBJECTIVE:

Applies knowledge about immunization to the care of infants and children.

QUESTION:

Which of these conditions in a 15-month-old infant would be a CONTRAINDICATION to the administration of measles-mumps-rubella (MMR) vaccine?

* 1. Allergy to eggs.
2. Allergy to cow's milk.
3. Sickle cell trait.
4. Iron-deficiency anemia.

A MULTIPLE-CHOICE QUESTION TO AN OBJECTIVE

OBJECTIVE:

Selects appropriate toys for the age and developmental level of children.

QUESTION:

Of the following toys, the one which best meets the safety and developmental needs of a normal 3-month-old infant is

* 1. a hanging mobile.
2. a hanging crib gym.
3. a colorful rubber ball.
4. a colorful giraffe-in-the-box.

A MULTIPLE-CHOICE QUESTION TO AN OBJECTIVE

OBJECTIVE:

Describe the effects of diarrhea on fluid and electrolyte balance in an infant.

QUESTION:

Susie, 8 months old, is brought to the emergency room with a history of diarrhea for the past 12 hours. In addition to irritability, an early sign of dehydration is

1. the absence of tears.
2. a loss of weight.
3. the flushing of skin.
* 4. a decrease in the number of urine-soaked diapers.
5. the presence of petit mal or grand mal convulsions.

A MULTIPLE-CHOICE QUESTION TO AN OBJECTIVE

OBJECTIVE:

Differentiates between appropriate and inappropriate emergency first aid for poisoning.

QUESTION:

A next-door neighbor comes running into your home with her child stating that the child just swallowed a quantity of toilet bowl cleaner. If all of the following products are available, which one would it be best to give the child immediately?

* 1. Milk.
2. Toast.
3. Syrup of Ipecac.
4. A carbonated drink.

A MULTIPLE-CHOICE QUESTION TO AN OBJECTIVE

OBJECTIVE:

Provide anticipatory guidance regarding the nutritional needs of well children.

SITUATION:

Susan Heald, Mrs. Heald's only child, is 12 months old when she is brought back to the well child clinic. Her weight and height are within the normal range for her age.

QUESTION:

In the conference with Mrs. Heald, the anticipatory guidance relevant to nutrition that should be included is that

1. Susan will probably need to be fed for the next few months.
* 2. Susan's appetite will probably decrease within the next six months.
3. Susan's acceptance of a wide variety of new foods will now be evident.
4. Susan will need an increasing amount of supplementary vitamins during the next two years.

A MULTIPLE-CHOICE QUESTION TO AN OBJECTIVE

OBJECTIVE:

Recognize appropriate nursing interventions when caring for an adolescent with a head injury.

SITUATION:

Craig Towner, 13 years old, is admitted to the hospital soon after sustaining a head injury when he was hit by a car while riding his bicycle. He is conscious.

QUESTION:

Based on the information provided about Craig, three of the following nursing interventions are appropriate. Which one is CONTRAINDICATED?

1. Keeping the siderails on his bed up at all times.
2. Assessing and documenting his neurological status every 15 to 30 minutes.
3. * Administering meperidine (Demerol) 35 mg q 4 h prn for pain, if ordered.
4. Notifying the physician of any change in his level of consciousness.

OBJECTIVE:

Identify the behaviors associated with hospitalization of children at all ages and developmental levels.

SITUATION:

See previous page

QUESTION:

Which of the following behaviors is Craig most likely to exhibit during his hospitalization?

* 1. Fails to comply with the treatment plan.
2. Reacts to parental separation by crying.
3. Demonstrates little regard for modesty.
4. Avoids forming relationships with his peers on the unit.

A MULTIPLE-CHOICE QUESTION TO AN OBJECTIVE

OBJECTIVE:

Identify the changes in vital signs that are indicative of increasing intracranial pressure.

QUESTION:

Which of the following changes in vital signs occurs early and indicates increasing intracranial pressure?

1. Narrowing pulse pressure, decreasing pulse rate, and increasing respiratory rate.
2. Narrowing pulse pressure, increasing pulse rate, and decreasing respiratory rate.

* 3. Widening pulse pressure, decreasing pulse rate, and decreasing respiratory rate.

4. Widening pulse pressure, increasing pulse rate, and increasing respiratory rate.

THE USE OF CLIENT SITUATIONS IN EXAMINATIONS

In the review of countless examinations over the years, I have found that the preponderance of multiple-choice questions are individual items. Occasionally, a faculty member may write two or three items based on the same client. One reason this practice probably exists is that it is easier to write individual items. However, in the real world clients have a variety of problems as well as a variety of normal functions. If we want our students to deal with clients holisticly, then perhaps we would be wise to focus our teaching as well as our evaluation procedures on the total client. One good way of following through on this concept is to develop client situations that mimic the real world of practice. A situation can be developed that begins with admission to the hospital and follows the client through discharge from the hospital and for a period of time at home. In other instances, situations can be developed that exclude the hospital and focus on an out-patient clinic, a well-child clinic, a mental health clinic, nursery school, camp or the like. Many questions can be asked about normal growth and development, physiology, psychological development, nutritional needs and all of the other content we include in our courses all related to an individual or a family. How much more meaningful this is likely to be for students! When asked, students have said that they relate to such situations, that the clients seem "real," and that they are more like actual practice.

A question often asked is how many questions should be included in a typical situation. The answer to that is--it all depends. To begin with, part of the answer to that question relates to the test blueprint and how many questions or what percentage of the test you elected to devote to the subject, content and/or objectives. In some instances you may want only four questions (for an area that is not very common) while for another topic such as normal pregnancy you may want to include 15 or 20 questions. It is a good idea to remember, however, that too many questions on a client may be cumbersome--you forget what happened at the beginning of the situation. In other instances, the students may lose interest.

When writing situations, "feed" in the bits and pieces of information that are necessary for answering the question or questions that follow. Although it may make it more interesting to read, do not include extraneous material because it may confuse the student, in addition to increasing reading time. There are instances, however, when you may wish to include a lot of data, if part of the purpose of the question is to sort out relevant data from irrelevant data. In general, typical multiple-choice situations should only include pertinent information. By building the situation as you progress, it is helpful to think of real clients and what happens to them in the course of, for example, their hospitalization. If one follows this advice, most of the needs of a client can be addressed, as well as relevant symptoms, pathophysiology, prognosis, and the like.

The sample client situations that follow illustrate many of the points mentioned above.

ORIGINAL SITUATION

Lucy Peanuts is a 4-year-old caucasian female who, until 2 months ago, was healthy. She subsequently developed a low grade fever (99°F. p.r.) and a cold, became very tired and chilly, where she was never intolerant to temperature.

Lucy's siblings, ages 1 and 3, also had intermittent colds, before Lucy evidenced these symptoms. Mrs. Peanuts delayed bringing Lucy to the doctor until the tiredness became chronic and Lucy looked pale and developed back and joint pains.

Dr. Schulz examined Lucy in the ER and noted; a thin pale, female, lethargic and irritable during examination. Her vital signs are as follows: T: 100.2°F., P: 164, R: 42; BP: 115/85. He also made the following notes; Enlarged cervical and inguinal lymph nodes; multiple ecchymosis and petechiae on her trunk and extremities; and multiple white papular lesions over mucosa and tongue with bleeding tissues in the corners of her mouth.

The laboratory data follows;

Hct 21% vol/100 ml	Hgb 7 Gm/100 ml.
WBC 2400	Lymphs 51%
Bands 10%	Blasts 1%
Polys 37%	Monos 1%
Platelets 33,500/cu mm	

Impression: Acute Lymphoblastic Leukemia

Dr. Schulz orders the follows;

1. Bed rest
2. Clear fluids
3. Protective isolation
4. IV 2½% Dextrose in Saline at 45 ml/hr.
5. Tylenol gr V p.o. or p.r. q 4-6 hours for temp. over 101.4°F.
6. Methotrexate 2.5 mgm p.o. t.i.d.
7. Prednisone 40 mgm, q.d. in 3 divided doses

1. The next step in treating Lucy is to perform a lumbar puncture. The LP revealed 490 WBC with 98% monocytes. Nursing intervention should stress
   * * A. preparing Lucy for the pain of the procedure.
   * B. instructing Lucy to lie flat for 12 hours.
   * C. allowing Lucy to play with needles and syringes.
   * D. watching for bleeding every two hours.

REVISED VERSION

1. A 4-year-old girl is admitted to the hospital for diagnostic tests. She is alert and responsive. Among the tests ordered for her is a lumbar puncture. Which of the following nursing interventions is most important in relation to this test?
   * * A. Preparing her for the pain of the procedure.
   * B. Allowing her to play with needle and syringe prior to the procedure.
   * C. Instructing her to lie flat for at least 12 hours following the procedure.
   * D. Observing her for bleeding following the procedure.

DISCUSSION

Although the "story" about Lucy and her family is interesting to read and although we may present such content in class for the purpose of discussion in the teaching/learning process, it is completely inappropriate in this situation. To begin with, there was only one question asked about the situation. Secondly, it is not good practice to use comic strip names or made up ones such as Mrs. Gastro Enteroscopy. Test taking is serious business and should be treated accordingly. I believe there is a time and place for humor but it is unrelated to examinations. Students seem to identify better with situations involving a client with a real name and a ready made supply can be found in a telephone directory. I have found that combining the first name of one with the surname of another works well. Be careful, however, of names in the news!

In the actual test question, the second sentence in the stem is out of place. The result of the lumbar puncture is given before the test was done! Note that the intended correct answer is preparing her for the procedure.

If it is necessary to develop a lengthy situation, make sure that adequate use is made of the data by writing a series of questions. In some instances, it is necessary to include data that is irrelevant as well as data that is relevant. In this instance, students may be asked to sort out the relevant from the irrelevant information.

In the typical situational-type format, data is included as necessary to answer the questions that follow. As a result, pieces of data and/or information are fed into the situation as appropriate. You unfold the situation as you follow a patient through his hospitalization or illness or stay in a convalescent home. Examples of this format follow.

SAMPLE CLIENT SITUATION--MEDICAL NURSING

Mrs. Helen Wills, 23 years old, has had diabetes mellitus for 10 years. When she is brought to the hospital by her mother, she is unconscious.

1. The nurse in the emergency room obtains the following vital signs: Blood pressure 130/88; temperature 99° F. by rectum; pulse 120; respirations 34. It has been established that Mrs. Wills takes 30 U. of NPH insulin daily. Based on the above data, the nurse should first
   - * 1. establish a patent airway for her.
   - 2. administer the 30 U. of NPH insulin subcutaneously.
   - 3. catheterize her for daily urine checks.
   - 4. start an intravenous on her with 1,000 cc of 5% dextrose in water.

2. After assessing Mrs. Wills and notifying the physician, the next action by the nurse should be to
   - 1. insert a foley catheter.
   - 2. give any prescribed insulin.
   - 3. obtain a history from the client's mother.
   - * 4. prepare to administer a hyperglycemic agent intravenously.

3. Mrs. Wills is to receive 30 U. of insulin intravenously. Of the following types of insulin, the only one that can be administered intravenously is
   - 1. NPH.
   - 2. Lente.
   - * 3. Regular.
   - 4. Protamine Zinc.

Mrs. Wills regains consciousness and is transferred to a medical unit.

4. At 10:00 A.M. on the morning after admission, the nurse finds Mrs. Wills confused and irritable and she is sweating. Which of these actions should the nurse take first?
   1. Check her vital signs.
   2. Obtain a urine specimen.
   3. Smell her breath for acetone.
   * 4. Give her sweetened orange juice.

After receiving appropriate therapy, Mrs. Wills recovers.

5. The nurse plans to teach Mrs. Wills how to avoid a recurrence of the complication. Three of the following preventive measures should be emphasized by the nurse. Which one is the <u>EXCEPTION</u>?
   1. Adherence to her diet.
   2. Daily testing of urine for sugar and acetone.
   3. Early reporting of signs and symptoms of infection.
   * 4. Avoidance of social activities involving crowds.

One week later, Mrs. Wills is packing to go home. She received NPH insulin at 7:30 A.M.

6. At 1:30 P.M., Mrs. Wills says to the nurse, "I feel funny." She appears pale and diaphoretic. Which of these initial responses would be best?
   1. "Did you eat all of your lunch?"
   2. "I will prepare your insulin now."
   * 3. "Let me get you some orange juice with sugar in it."
   4. "Lie down. I will need to take your blood pressure."

<u>NOTE</u>: It is desirable to use a different pitch or type style for the history or situation between questions. It alerts the student to the difference between the situation and the items.

SAMPLE CLIENT SITUATION--MEDICAL NURSING

Mrs. Hilda Wilde, 24 years old, has had diabetes mellitus for 10 years. When she is brought to the hospital emergency room, she is unconscious. Her mother is with her. It has been established that her diabetes has been controlled with insulin.

1. Which of these nursing interventions would be most appropriate for Mrs. Wilde initially?
   1. Notify the physician of her arrival.
   2. Establish an intravenous with normal saline.
   3. Check her urine for sugar and acetone.
   * 4. Ask her mother the type and time of her last insulin administration.

2. Based on the initial assessment of Mrs. Wilde, the nurse is unable to determine if the patient is in diabetic coma or insulin shock. Which of the following drugs or solutions should the nurse anticipate being administered to the client first?
   1. Glucagon.
   2. Regular insulin.
   3. 5% dextrose in water.
   * 4. 50% dextrose in water

3. Mrs. Wilde's initial blood sugar is 850 mg/100 ml. Which of these insulin preparations will lower her blood sugar the fastest?
   1. NPH.
   2. Lente.
   * 3. Regular.
   4. Ultralente.

Mrs. Wilde regains consciousness and is transferred to a medical unit. She has been receiving fluids intravenously.

4. Between 9:00 A.M. and 10:00 A.M. Mrs. Wilde's urinary output is 10 cc. What should the nurse do first?
    1. Increase her intravenous flow rate.
    * 2. Report her output to the physician.
    3. Collect her urine for another hour.
    4. Check the specific gravity of her urine.

5. When making rounds, the nurse finds Mrs. Wilde pale and diaphoretic. Mrs. Wilde says that she feels tremulous. The most appropriate nursing intervention initially would be to
    1. test her urine.
    * 2. give her orange juice.
    3. check her vital signs.
    4. administer insulin to her.

Three days later, Mrs. Wilde is sufficiently recovered to be concerned about the prevention of ketoacidosis in the future. The nurse initiates a teaching plan.

6. In order to assist Mrs. Wilde to manage her blood sugar levels, it is essential for the nurse to assess three of the following areas. Which one is <u>NOT</u> essential?
    * 1. Sleep pattern.
    2. Dietary habits.
    3. Insulin dosage.
    4. Activity schedule.

In order to round out the sample of content that assesses knowledge pertaining to diabetes mellitus, you may wish to include one or more individual items. The following question is an example of the type you may wish to include.

Individual Item.

Mr. Peal is a 25-year-old insulin-dependent diabetic who is employed as an accountant. One Saturday morning after several hours of gardening, he goes into his house to lie down before lunch. His wife hears a thud and finds Mr. Peal uncounscious. Before taking Mr. Peal to the emergency room, which of the following actions, if any, should Mrs. Peal take?

1. Give him 1 milligram of glucagon.
2. Give him 5 units of regular insulin.
3. Give him 4 ounces of orange juice.

* 4. None of them.

SAMPLE CLIENT SITUATION--SURGICAL NURSING

Mr. Sam Babson, a 35-year-old truck driver, has had a peptic ulcer for several years. He is admitted to the hospital soon after having a large emesis of what he described as "dark blood."

1. During the admission procedure, Mr. Babson vomits bright red blood. The initial action should be to
    1. give him an emesis basin.
    2. turn his head to one side.
    3. collect a specimen for analysis.
    * 4. take his vital signs.

2. Which of these understandings should the nurse have in order to assess the emesis?
    1. It is vomitus and comes from the lung.
    2. It comes from the lung and may be of coffee-ground consistency.
    * 3. It may be of coffee-ground consistency and comes from the stomach.
    4. It comes from the stomach and is hemoptysis.

3. The nurse collects the following data from Mr. Babson;

    Blood pressure 90/70
    Pulse 120 and thready
    Respirations 30 and shallow
    Skin pale, cold and clammy

    Based on the above data, how should Mr. Babson be positioned?
    1. Elevate the head of his bed only.
    2. Elevate the foot of his bed only.
    3. Elevate his torso only.
    * 4. Flatten both the head and foot of his bed.

4. Mr. Babson is scheduled for a barium swallow in the morning and the nurse gives him the appropriate dietary instruction. Which of these comments by Mr. Babson on the morning he is scheduled for the barium swallow would indicate that he understood the instructions given to him?
   1. "I ate all my supper last night."
   2. "I refused supper because I knew I wasn't supposed to eat."
   * 3. "I have had nothing to eat or drink since midnight."
   4. "I had a liquid diet for breakfast this morning."

5. Mr. Babson has had no further episodes of emesis. He is placed on a regular diet but has been refusing meals and is drinking only small amounts of fluids. Observation of Mr.Babson reveals poor skin turgor, dry cracked lips, and concentrated urine with 100 cc of output in the last 8 hours. Which of these actions should be taken first?
   1. Apply lemon and glycerine to Mr. Babson's lips.
   * 2. Assess Mr. Babson's preferences for fluids.
   3. Calculate an accurate intake for the previous 8 hours.
   4. Give the patient 100 cc of a nourishing fluid.

Mr. Babson is scheduled for a gastrojejunostomy.

6. Which of these positions is appropriate for Mr. Babson while he is on the operating table?
   1. Jackknife.
   2. Lithotomy.
   * 3. Dorsal recumbent.
   4. Semi-Fowler's.

SAMPLE CLIENT SITUATION--ORTHOPEDIC NURSING

Mrs. Molly Blake, a 74-year-old housewife, is admitted to the hospital after having fallen down a flight of stairs in her home. She has a right trochanteric fracture.

1. Mrs. Blake complains of severe pain in her right hip. In assessing Mrs. Blake's pain, which of the following signs and symptoms would indicate stimulation of the sympathetic nervous system?

    1. Decreased pulse rate and elevated blood pressure.
    2. Decreased pulse rate and decreased respirations.
    3. Increased pulse rate and decreased respirations.

    * 4. Increased pulse rate and elevated blood pressure.

Mrs. Blake has an open reduction,internal fixation of the right hip.

2. Following surgery, how should the nurse position Mrs. Blake's right leg while she is in supine position?

    * 1. Abduction with knee flexion.

    2. Adduction with knee extension.
    3. External rotation with knee extension.
    4. Internal rotation with knee flexion.

3. To help prevent pneumonia in Mrs. Blake, which of the following actions by the nurse is essential?

    1. Turn her from side to side every 2 hours.

    * 2. Assist her to cough and deep breathe every 2 hours.

    3. Maintain her fluid intake at 3,000 cc in a 24-hour period.
    4. Keep the head of her bed elevated at a 45° angle at all times.

Mrs. Blake is progressing favorably and she is able to ambulate with the assistance of a walker.

4. The nurse's plan of care for Mrs. Blake should include three of the following actions. Which one is the EXCEPTION?

   1. Consult with her physician regarding discharge planning.
   2. Consult with personnel in the hospital home care program about her status.
   3. Initiate a referral to the community nursing service.
   - * 4. Initiate arrangements for placement in a nursing home.

SAMPLE CLIENT SITUATION--GENITOURINARY NURSING

Mr. Lou Green, 65 years old, is admitted to the hospital with symptoms of acute urinary retention.

1. The physician orders that Mr. Green be catheterized immediately using a French catheter.The bladder is still distended after 800 cc of urine has drained. The most appropriate nursing action would be to

   * 1. remove the catheter and notify the physician.
   2. clamp the catheter for ½ hour before continuing to empty the bladder.
   3. permit the catheter to continue draining by connecting it to gravity drainage.
   4. connect the catheter to gravity drainage and apply gentle pressure over the suprapubic area.

Mr. Green is discharged but is readmitted the following day with similar complaints.

2. An indwelling foley catheter is to be inserted in Mr. Green. The first step in initiating the appropriate teaching is to

   1. explain how the catheter will be inserted.
   2. explain the physical feelings he may experience.
   3. ask if he knows how to care for a foley catheter.
   * 4. ask if he has ever had a foley catheter inserted before.

3. Appropriate nursing care of Mr. Green's indwelling catheter includes

   1. changing his catheter q.o.d.
   2. irrigating his catheter q.4.h.
   3. clamping the catheter when he ambulates.
   * 4. positioning the drainage bag below his bladder.

Mr. Green has a transurethral resection (TUR) of the prostate.

4. When Mr. Green has been returned to his room following surgery, he sees the bloody drainage in his urine drainage bag and expresses alarm. Which of the following actions should be taken by the nurse?

    1. Notify Mr. Green's physician immediately.
    2. Irrigate Mr. Green's retention catheter.
    * 3. Explain to Mr. Green that the occurrence is an expected one.
    4. Check the physician's orders and administer any appropriate medication.

AN ALTERNATE APPROACH TO TESTING THE CONTENT IN QUESTION NUMBER 1 ON THE PRECEDING PAGE FOLLOWS.

1. The physician orders the insertion of a French catheter. During the catheterization procedure, the nurse should take 3 of the following actions. Which one is the <u>EXCEPTION</u>?

    1. Use sterile technique.
    * 2. Attach the catheter to drainage.
    3. Observe the color, consistency, and odor of the urine.
    4. Check for resistance during the insertion of the catheter.

SAMPLE CLIENT SITUATION--OBSTETRIC NURSING

Mrs. Stella Ford, 34 years old, comes to the prenatal clinic for the first time in the sixth month of her pregnancy. She reports having had frequent headaches for a week. The Fords have two other children. Laboratory tests yield the following data:

A. Negative VDRL
B. Glucose 110 mg/100 ml
C. HCT 25%
D. HGB 9 gm
E. WBC 8,500 per cu mm

1. Based on the laboratory results, which of the following nursing interventions is most appropriate for Mrs. Ford?

   1. Assess the client's knowledge of venereal disease prevention.
   2. Contact the physician regarding the need for antibiotic therapy.
   3. Instruct the client in how to collect a double-voided urine specimen.
   * 4. Provide dietary instructions on foods high in iron.

Mrs. Ford returns to the clinic in her seventh month of pregnancy. Because she is toxic, she is admitted to the hospital.

2. All of the following rooms are available. To which one should Mrs. Ford be admitted?

   1. A private room overlooking the park.
   * 2. A quiet, darkened private room.
   3. A darkened semi-private room shared with a mother whose infant was stillborn.
   4. A cheerful, semi-private room shared with a new mother.

3. Mrs. Ford has a convulsion. All of the following actions should be taken. Which one should the nurse take first?

   1. Call for assistance.
   2. Check the fetal heart tones.
   3. Notify her doctor.
   * 4. Protect her from injury.

Mrs. Ford has been receiving magnesium sulfate ($MgSO_4$) for the past 24 hours.

4. Before administering the next dose of magnesium sulfate to Mrs. Ford, it is essential for the nurse to assess her reflexes and

   1. blood pressure and pulse.
   2. pulse and temperature.
   3. temperature and respirations.
   * 4. respirations and blood pressure.

Mrs. Ford's condition improves and she is discharged. She is readmitted to the obstetric unit in active labor in the 37th week of gestation. External fetal monitoring has been initiated.

5. The nurse observes 2 successive late decelerations. In addition to notifying the physician, it would be most appropriate for the nurse to take which of these actions?

   1. Elevate the head of her bed and administer oxygen by mask.
   2. Lower the head of her bed and check her vital signs.
   * 3. Have her turn on her left side and administer oxygen by mask.
   4. Have her turn on her right side and check her vital signs.

SAMPLE CLIENT SITUATION--OBSTETRIC NURSING

Mrs. Joan Taylor, 25 years old, comes to the antepartal clinic after missing a menstrual period. A pregnancy test is performed and the result is positive.

1. The hormone that is the basis of a positive pregnancy test is

    1. estrogen.
    2. progesterone.
    3. prostiglandin.

    * 4. chorionic gonadatropin.

2. If Mrs. Taylor's last menstrual period was June 14, 1983, her expected date of confinement will be

    1. March 7, 1984.

    * 2. March 21, 1984.

    3. April 7, 1984.
    4. April 21, 1984.

Mrs. Taylor returns to the clinic when she is 8 months pregnant. She tells the nurse that she has had no care since her initial visit to the clinic.

3. Which of the following questions should be asked of Mrs. Taylor initially?

    * 1. "How have things been going for you?"

    2. "Were you unable to get to the clinic?"
    3. "Why haven't you had medical care lately?"
    4. "What prevented you from coming to the clinic?"
    5. "Have you been feeling all right since you were here last?"

Mrs. Taylor spontaneously delivers a 4 lb. 2 oz. boy.

4. Baby Boy Taylor's Apgar score is 7 at 1 minute. Such a score is indicative of

    1. guarded status.

    * 2. satisfactory status.

    3. immenent circulatory collapse.
    4. impending respiratory collapse.

SAMPLE CLIENT SITUATION--OBSTETRIC NURSING

Mrs. Becky Temple, 21 years old, is admitted to the hospital in active labor. This is the Temples' first baby. Mrs. Temple attended preparation for childbirth classes. Mr. Temple will stay with his wife during labor.

1. Which of the following actions should be taken first when Mrs. Temple is admitted to the labor room?

    1. Ascertain her E.D.C.
    * 2. Obtain her vital signs.
    3. Palpate her abdomen for fetal position.
    4. Find out if she plans to breast-feed her infant.

2. After the admission procedure is completed, which of these measures would be most appropriate?

    1. Showing the Temples relaxation techniques.
    * 2. Finding out what the Temples know about the labor and delivery process.
    3. Allowing the Temples time to be together without unnecessary interference.
    4. Letting the Temples know that the nurse will stay with them throughout labor and delivery.

Mrs. Temple delivers an 8 lb. 4 oz. male infant without complication.

3. Immediately after the infant is delivered, which of these actions is indicated?

    1. Administer Deladumone.
    2. Estimate her blood loss.
    * 3. Check her blood pressure.
    4. Wait for delivery of the placenta.

Mrs. Temple is brought to the postpartum recovery room. Her husband and infant are with her.

4. Which of these measures is indicated at this time?

    * 1. Showing the Temples how to hold their infant.
    2. Teaching Mrs. Temple how to do perineal care.
    3. Helping Mrs. Temple to breast-feed her infant.
    4. Demonstrating how to conduct an appraisal of their infant.

SAMPLE CLIENT SITUATION--PEDIATRIC NURSING

James Avis is born after 36 weeks gestation. At birth, a systolic heart murmur is heard over the pulmonary artery.

1. At birth, the premature infant should be handled as little as possible because handling subjects him to which of the following conditions?
    1. Trauma
    2. Infection
    3. Exhaustion
    4. Kernicterus

   A. 1 and 2
   B. 2 and 4
   * C. 1, 2, and 3
   D. 1, 3, and 4

Twenty-four hours after birth, he develops respiratory distress syndrome with severe central cyanosis.

2. In order to determine if the central cyanosis is pulmonary or cardiac in origin, he should be placed in
   A. a thermal-neutral environment for observation.
   B. semi-Fowler's position and his nasopharynx suctioned.
   C. 40% oxygen and stimulated to cry.
   * D. 100% oxygen and have arterial blood gases drawn.

Forty-eight hours later, the respiratory distress abates but the cyanosis persists for several days. It is determined that the cyanosis is cardiac in origin.

3. Although James recovers from the episode of respiratory distress, the effect of the episode on his prognosis is probably
   A. an increase in the frequency of respiratory problems.
   * B. no increase in the frequency of respiratory problems.
   C. typical frequency but greater severity of respiratory problems.
   D. an increased frequency but typical severity of respiratory problems.

A cardiac catheterization and angiocardiogram are done and James is diagnosed as having moderate interatrial septal defect.

4. Following the cardiac catheterization, nursing intervention should include observation at least every 30 minutes for

* * A. peripheral pulse rates and persistent cardiac arrhythmias.
* B. peripheral pulse rates and loss of consciousness.
* C. elevation of temperature and persistent cardiac arrhythmias.
* D. elevation of temperature and loss of consciousness.

5. James has difficulty with feeding as do most infants with congenital heart disease. He is likely to feed with less difficulty if

* A. his formula is warmed prior to feeding.
* B. his diaper is changed prior to feeding.
* C. he is burped after every two or three ounces.
* * D. he is fed small amounts at a time.

When James is 10 days old, the cyanosis subsides and he is to be discharged to await corrective surgery.

6. In preparation for James' discharge, the nurse teaches his parents the signs of congestive heart failure. Which of the following signs should be included?

   1. Excessive sweating
   2. Excessive crying
   3. Difficult breathing
   4. Abdominal distention

* A. 1 and 3
* B. 1 and 4
* C. 2 and 4
* * D. 3 and 4

When James is 3 years old, he is brought to the pediatric clinic.

7. Mrs. Avis asks the nurse how much activity James should be allowed to have. Which of the following statements contains the information that should be given to James' mother?

   A. James should be watched for the occurrence of paroxysmal dyspneic attacks.

   B. James should not be allowed to engage in strenuous activities such as riding a tricycle.

   * C. A child of this age is usually self-limiting in his activities and needs no special limits.

   D. A child of this age needs guidance in everyday activities so that he will learn how to pace himself.

SAMPLE CLIENT SITUATION--PEDIATRIC NURSING

Linda Webb, 4 months old, is admitted to the hospital with the diagnosis of bronchial pneumonia. Her temperature is 103.6° F. by rectum.

1. Which of these patterns of pulse and respiratory rates is likely to correlate most closely with Linda's temperature?

   1. Pulse 86; respirations 24.
   2. Pulse 102; respirations 30.
   3. Pulse 120; respirations 40.

   * 4. Pulse 180; respirations 52.

2. Which of these independent actions should the nurse take initially to lower Linda's temperature?

   1. Give her 8 ounces of iced apple juice.

   * 2. Give her a tepid sponge bath.

   3. Place her in a cool mist tent.
   4. Administer 0.3 cc of Tylenol p.o. stat.

3. In planning Linda's care while she is acutely ill, the following actions should be taken in what sequence?

   A. Suction her.
   B. Feed her.
   C. Allow her to rest.

1. A, B, C

* 2. A, C, B

3. B, C, A
4. C, A, B

SAMPLE CLIENT SITUATION--PSYCHIATRIC NURSING

Mrs. Trudy Hill, 50 years old, has become increasingly depressed and agitated since her husband died a year ago and her daughter married and left her. She now moans and cries almost constantly, and accuses herself of great "sins." After being found with her wrists cut by a razor blade, she is admitted to a psychiatric unit , following treatment of her wounds.

1. All of the following nursing interventions are important when Mrs. Hill is admitted to her unit. Which one should be done first?

    1. The establishment of a 1:1 relationship.
    * 2. The assessment of her current suicide risk.
    3. The examination of her wrist wounds for infection.
    4. The evaluation of her environment for hazards.

2. When the nurse enters Mrs. Hill's room, Mrs. Hill is wringing her hands and moaning, "It's all my fault. I killed my husband." Which of the following initial responses would be the most therapeutic?

    1. "Would you like to talk?"
    2. "You believe that you killed your husband?"
    3. "I don't believe that you killed your husband."
    * 4. "I can see that you are upset. Let's talk about it."

3. Twenty-four hours later when the nurse enters Mrs. Hill's room, Mrs. Hill says, "I can't believe I tried to cut my wrists. Surely you don't think I'll try that again!" The most appropriate response by the nurse would be

    1. "Oh, I'm sure glad you said that!"
    2. "No, I'm not sure you wouldn't try to do that again."
    3. "Most people who try suicide once, may try again."
    * 4. "What makes you believe that you wouldn't try it again?"

4. In the first few days of Mrs. Hill's hospitalization, which of these nursing actions should receive priority?

   * 1. Checking Mrs. Hill at frequent, staggered intervals.

   2. Contracting with Mrs. Hill for daily 50-minute counseling sessions.

   3. Providing Mrs. Hill with structured daily activities.

   4. Interviewing Mrs. Hill for her current suicide ideation.

SOME GUIDELINES FOR WRITING COMBINATION-TYPE ITEMS

Sample Question

Signs of dehydration in young infants include which of the following?

A. Hot, dry skin
B. Poor skin turgor
C. Sunken fontanelles
D. Scanty, concentrated urine

1. A and C
2. B and D
3. A, B, and D
4. All of them

Discussion

For the sample question presented above, suppose I had these options instead:

1. C only
2. A and C
3. B, C, and D
4. All of them

You should note that choice C appears in each of the options which is permissible since one of the options is "C only". However, there are other times when this practice is undesirable. Consider, for example, the following set of options:

1. A and C
2. B and C
3. B, C, and D
4. All of them

In this last example, C serves no function at all since it occurs in each option along with one or more letters. In this instance, the C is a given and tests nothing.

In a combination-type multiple-choice question with 3 choices it is possible to have a set of options like this:

1. A only
2. B only
3. A and B
4. B and C

It is also possible to use as options "none of them" and/or "all of them". A word of caution in relation to "all of them"--faculty tend to overuse this choice especially as the correct answer and students soon detect this tendency. In 4-option questions when "all of them" is offered, it should only be correct about 25% of the time.

When the choice "none of them" is offered, it is necessary to include two words in the stem of the question to make this option plausible, namely, if any.

Which of the following symptoms, if any, etc.

These two words, if any, give credence to the fact that none of the symptoms (or whatever) may be present or may occur. When "none of them" is offered as an option, the same practice should be observed as with "all of them", namely, that it should be correct only about 25% of the time. This statement should also indicate that it should be incorrect most of the time. Faculty seem to avoid making it correct even some of the time.

Combination-type multiple-choice questions can be used very successfully in examinations if some of these pointers are borne in mind in their initial construction. Another point to be mentioned is the fact that no question can test everything. It is a far better practice to construct several items rather than expect one question to assess several important points.Of course, there are possibilities for testing more than one point in a question. One example that comes to mind is cause and effect questions. In the examples that follow in this chapter you will find examples of such questions.

SAMPLE FORMAT FOR COMBINATION-TYPE MULTIPLE-CHOICE QUESTIONS

1. Which of these symptoms commonly occur in diabetes mellitus?

    1. Loss of weight
    2. Excessive thirst
    3. Increased appetite
    4. Increased urination
    5. Frequent skin infections

  A. 1 and 2
  B. 3, 4, and 5
* C. 2, 3, 4, and 5
  D. All of them

2. Which of these measures are included in the treatment of allergies?

    A. Immunizing when possible
    B. Having psychiatric intervention
    C. Separating the individual from allergens
    D. Relieving the effects of allergic responses

  1. A, B, and C
  2. A, B, and D
  3. A, C, and D
  4. B, C, and D
  5. All of the above

NOTE: Use either letters <u>or</u> numbers for options, not both. What you use may be dictated by the type of answer sheet and/or scoring equipment you have access to. Options for combination-type items should be the same as the single-option type.

Although I believe a variety of combinations is desirable, I should mention that some testing agencies use the same set of combinations in each of their questions.

ORIGINAL VERSION

An elderly client with dry skin or a critically ill client may not need a full bath each day. According to Lewis, a partial bath would include the following:

1. washing face, hands, axilla, back, perineal area, and massaging the back.
2. washing face, arms, chest, and massaging the back.
3. washing the face, hands, arms, feet, back, perineal area, and massaging the back.
4. washing any body part which is soiled or has an offensive odor.

REVISED VERSION

According to Lewis, in addition to massaging the back, a partial bath includes washing which of the following areas?

A. Arms
B. Axilla
C. Back
D. Chest
E. Face
F. Feet
G. Hands
H. Perineum

1. A, D, and E
2. A, B, D, and F
* 3. B, C, E, G, and H
4. A, C, E, F, G, and H

COMMENTS: Generally I do not advocate so many choices in an item such as this, but since the options are short (one word), it should be easy to respond. The first sentence of the stem in the original item is a "teaching" sentence and is unnecessary. I put "massaging the back" in the stem of the revised item because it was longer than the other choices. In doing so, it may make the item a little harder. I believe the revision is an improvement over the original.

ORIGINAL VERSION

J. Doe, UMNS, is teaching his client how to floss teeth using the procedure described in Lewis. He instructs her to:

1. wrap the floss on her middle finger.
2. have her thumb to the outside for the upper teeth.
3. floss between upper and lower back teeth.
4. 1 and 3 only.
5. All of the above.

REVISED VERSION

According to Lewis, how should teeth be flossed?

1. Wrap the floss around the middle finger
2. Floss between the upper and lower back teeth
3. For the upper teeth, the thumb should be on the outside

A. 1 only
B. 2 only
C. 1 and 2
D. 1 and 3
* E. All of them

COMMENTS: In the original item, options 4 and 5 are inappropriate because single option multiple-choice format is being mixed with a combination-type one. I believe it is confusing to students. The stem was revised to include only necessary information. Whether a nursing student is doing it or an RN, the technique should be the same. Also "He instructs her to" is poor because he may instruct her to do any of the choices. However, we know how teeth should be flossed.

ORIGINAL VERSION

The early signs of a decubitus ulcer include:

1. pale, irritated skin followed by reddened skin
2. irritated and tender skin
3. extreme pain
4. small broken area 1-2 cm in size

A. 1, 2, and 3
B. 1 and 2
C. 1 and 3
D. 1, 2, and 4

REVISED VERSION

Which of the following signs and symptoms occur early in the development of decubitus ulcers?

1. Irritated and tender skin
2. Pale, irritated skin followed by reddened skin
3. A small, broken area of skin about 1 - 2 cm in size
4. Severe pain in and around the involved area of skin

* A. 1 and 2
B. 1 and 3
C. 2 and 4
D. 3 and 4

COMMENTS: With a combination-type item, the stem should be closed to reduce response time. In the options, 1 is included in each so is testing nothing, while the choice 4 is only used once. The word "skin" is included only in the correct answer--1 and 2,so provides a clue. In the revision, it was added to 3 and 4. In the original, options A through D are illogical and therefore, harder to find the answer.

NOTE: Do not use the question that follows along with this one since a clue is provided to the correct answer.

ORIGINAL VERSION

Potential complications that may arise from bedrest are:
1. decubitus ulcers
2. orthostatic hypotension
3. gastrointestinal disturbances
4. bleeding tendencies
A. 1, 3, 4
B. 1, 2, 3
C. 1, 2, 4
D. All of the above

REVISED VERSION

Which of the following complications may occur as a result of bedrest for a period of time?

1. Decubitus ulcers
2. Orthostatic hypotension
3. Gastrointestinal disturbances
4. Bleeding tendencies

A. 1 only
B. 1 and 2
* C. 1, 2, and 3
D. All of them

COMMENTS: The stem should be closed in a combination-type item and the choices should start with a capital letter. The spacing and format should be different for the numbers and the letters because it is very confusing as presented. I recommend that an "and" be used before the last choice in an option, e.g., 1, 2, and 3. It lets the student know that a piece of the option wasn't inadvertantly left off. Options A through D are illogically presented and choice 1 appears in each so is testing nothing. In the revised version, 1 is presented alone which then asks, "Is something besides 1 also correct?"

NOTE: This item should not be used with the preceding question because a clue is provided to the correct answer.

ORIGINAL VERSION

At 8:00 a.m. you take Mrs. Brown's vital signs. You obtain a blood pressure reading of 110/64 and a pulse rate of 74.

1. 110 is the systolic pressure
2. 110 is the diastolic pressure
3. 64 is the systolic pressure
4. 64 is the diastolic pressure
5. 46 is the pulse pressure
6. 46 is the pulse deficit
7. 74 is the pulse pressure

A. 1, 4, and 6
B. 2, 3, and 5
C. 1, 4, and 5
D. 2, 3, and 6
E. 1, 4, and 7

REVISED VERSION

A blood pressure of 110/64 and a pulse rate of 74 are obtained on a client. Which of the following statements are correct about these findings?

1. 46 is the pulse deficit
2. 46 is the pulse pressure
3. 64 is the diastolic pressure
4. 64 is the systolic pressure
5. 74 is the pulse pressure
6. 110 is the diastolic pressure
7. 110 is the systolic pressure

A. 1, 4, and 6
B. 1, , and 7
C. 2, 3, and 4
* D. 2, 3, and 7
E. 4, 5, and 6

COMMENTS: The original version does not ask a question--the student has to read all of the choices before assuming what is wanted. The time and the patient's name in the stem are irrelevant. In the revision, I ordered the choices from low (46) to high (110) and presented A through E logically. I used each of the choices two times except for 4 which is used three times. (In the original version, 7 was used only one time.)

ORIGINAL VERSION

Lactose deficiency:

1. is found in many infants.
2. results in the inability to absorb milk sugar.
3. results in flatulence, diarrhea and pain.
4. results in ketosis.
5. is a rare occurrence in adults.

A. 2, 3
B. 2, 4
C. All except 2
D. All of the above

REVISED VERSION

Which of these statements are true about lactose intolerance?

1. It is found in many infants.
2. It is a rare occurrence in adults.
3. It results in the inability to digest milk sugar.
4. It results in mental retardation.
5. It results in flatulence, diarrhea, and pain.

A. 2 and 3.
B. 1, 2, and 4.
* C. 1, 3, and 5.
D. All of the above.

COMMENTS: The stem is unacceptable because no problem is presented. The format is confusing because there is no distinction between the numbers and the letters. This item also illustrates one of the reasons why this type of item is abused--it deals with both occurrence and results. In validating the correct answer, I found the term "lactose intolerance" used rather than "lactose deficiency." In the original version, option C is stated poorly--the student must identify what is not stated before responding (a two-step process.)

SAMPLE COMBINATION-TYPE MULTIPLE-CHOICE QUESTIONS

1. Place the following events related to left ventricular failure after a myocardial infarction in the correct sequence.

    A. Pulmonary congestion
    B. Dilatation and hypertrophy
    C. Necrosis of a portion of the left ventricle
    D. Decreased functional capacity of the left ventricle

    1. B, D, C, A
    2. C, B, A, D
    3. C, D, B, A
    * 4. D, C, A, B

2. A client may react differently to pain for which of the following reasons?

    A. Various cultural expectations
    B. Past experiences with pain
    C. Variations in the cognitive perception of pain
    D. Differences in the physiological pain threshold

    1. D only.
    2. C and D.
    3. A, B, and C.
    * 4. All of them.

SAMPLE COMBINATION-TYPE MULTIPLE-CHOICE QUESTIONS

(MATERNITY NURSING)

1. Mechanisms which compensate for the low oxygen tension of umbilical vein blood include which of the following?

   A. Higher hematocrit

   B. Increased secretion of angiotensin

   C. Increased rate of blood flow in the fetal circulation

   D. Greater affinity of fetal red blood cells for oxygen

   1. C only
   2. B and D

   * 3. A, C, and D

   4. All of them

2. A pregnant woman develops signs and symptoms of severe preeclampsia at 40 weeks gestation. Which of the following combinations of signs and symptoms, if present, would indicate that this woman might become eclamptic?

   1. Frontal headaches, hemodilution, and hyporeflexia.
   2. Frontal headaches, generalized edema, and hyperreflexia

   * 3. Epigastric pain, hemoconcentration, and diplopia

   4. Epigastric pain, pedal edema, and CNS irritability

3. Which of the following statements are true of $MgSO_4$?

   A. It is a CNS depressant

   B. It lowers the blood pressure

   C. It should not be given if the respiratory rate is below 12/minute

   D. It should be given if the patient is hypereflexic

   1. A, B, and C
   2. A, B, and D
   3. A, C, and D

   * 4. B, C, and D

(NOTE: Question #3 might also be used in other clinical tests)

MATCHING ITEMS

There have been many criticisms levelled against matching items as well as many abuses in actual practice. One has only to look at some of the examples available. One example in a published text book with which I am familiar contained literally a whole page of choices in one question! Such an overt abuse in construction results in nothing more than an exercise in futility or one might say, simply a clerical task. The student gets lost in the morass and forgets the assignment.

Matching questions can be very useful in testing definitions, facts, meanings, interpretations, and the like. Diagrams, charts, figures, and drawings can also be used where the task for the student would be to, for example, match the corresponding name with a body part.

The following tips are offered to assist you in writing better matching questions. Some of them are intended to maximize the chances that a student will get the answers right if she or he has the requisite knowledge rather than because she or he is test-wise. The constructor of test questions must also be test-wise and avoid building into the test questions clues or cues that would assist the test-wise student to get the answers right in the absence of the necessary knowledge.

Guidelines for Writing the Sets of Questions

1. Head each of the columns with a word or phrase that accurately describes the choices that will follow. This practice will require discrimination on the student's part and will also assist the test writer to keep the set of choices homogeneous. In addition, it helps to define the task for the student. If you find it difficult to label the columns, more than likely you have a heterogeneous set.

2. Keep the list of choices confined to a maximum of 6 to 8. More than this amount makes it analogous to a guessing game rather than a test of knowledge. In addition, keeping the list of choices relatively short, makes it more than likely that the set will be homogeneous.

3. If one of the columns contains words or short phrases and the other column contains longer statements, have the students select their choices from the list that requires the least amount of reading.

4. Generally speaking, offer more choices than the statements with which they are to be matched. Several exceptions to this rule include: (1) when some of the choices are to be used more than once and (2) when there are only a limited number that can logically be offered (such as Normal and Abnormal or Increased and Decreased). The probability of a student's guessing correctly is reduced when there are more choices. In addition, it avoids giving the student a bonus point--that is, if there are 4 choices in each list, the student would automatically get the fourth one if she or he got the first three.

5. To reduce the amount of reading time and the amount of time necessary to find the correct answer, arrange the options in logical or numerical order, when appropriate. The student will then not need to read and reread excessively to select the correct answer (assuming she or he knows it). It is usually unnecessary to arrange choices alphabetically, especially if they are statements but short phrases and words could certainly be so ordered.

6. Be sure to indicate in the directions whether or not choices may be used more than once and whether or not all choices will be used. Incomplete instructions to the students can be frustrating not only to the students but also to the instructor when tests are returned to students and they criticize the test directions, using that as one reason for their poor performance on the test.

7. As with all tests and test questions, allow adequate space for typing the directions and questions to facilitate reading. Do not squeeze everything together and by all means, do not separate parts of the same question. Keep all parts of a question on the same page. If a drawing or diagram is to be used, this practice may not be possible. It may be necessary to include all of the diagrams, drawings and the like in a supplement that can be referred to as necessary or as a pull-out sheet. Be sure, however, to have students return all test materials after the testing session!

8. Indicate the number of points to be awarded for each option or question--probably following the directions would be as good as any place for doing this. If each test question, regardless of type of question, is to receive the same number of points, this can be included in the overall instructions at the beginning of the test.

9. The same directions may be used for the entire section dealing with matching questions unless, of course, different instructions are necessary. For example, in some instances you may state that choices may be used more than once and in other questions you may want them to be used one time only. Another instance of the need to have specific directions for each set is when you elect to include the titles of each column in the directions. I am more inclined to be specific in my directions since I believe it helps students to demonstrate their knowledge <u>because</u> the directions spell out the precise task. Most of the examples that follow illustrate my practice.

<u>Critique of the questions beginning on page 93</u>.

For each of the sets of questions, I have indicated at the bottom of the revised set the guidelines that were violated. In some instances, additional comments address specific problems and/or concerns.

SAMPLE DIRECTIONS FOR MATCHING QUESTIONS

It is very important to give examinee's the rules of the game. They need to know the basis upon which they are to match items. Can a choice be used more than once? Are all choices to be used? Are there times when more than one choice is appropriate?

Depending on the number and type of matching sets, it may be possible to use the same set of directions for all of the sets. In other circumstances, individual directions will need to be given for each set. My personal preference is for individual sets of directions because each of them can be tailor-made to fit the situation. The examples which follow present a variety of directions and circumstances.

Another factor that needs to be included in the directions is the number of points to be awarded for each item. This can generally be accomplished by including it at the end of the directions in parentheses, for example, (6 points). If all test questions are to be given equal credit, the instructions at the beginning of the test can reflect this.

Samples

DIRECTIONS: In the blank to the left of each event listed in Column A, write the letter next to the physician's name in Column B who is noted for that event. Each name in Column B may be used once or not at all.

DIRECTIONS: For each event in the column on the left, select the date in the right column on which this event occurred and mark the corresponding letter on the answer sheet. Each date is to be used only once. (4 points)

DIRECTIONS: For each of the medication orders in the column on the left, select the correct definition in the right column and insert the corresponding letter in the blank space. Each of the definitions may be used once or not at all.

DIRECTIONS: For each of the predisposing factors specific to either placenta previa or abruptio placentae, select the correct condition in the right column and insert the corresponding letter in the blank space. Each of the letters is to be used at least once and may be used more than once.

DIRECTIONS: Match the term in the right-hand column with the appropriate example in the left-hand column and insert the corresponding letter in the blank space. Each letter may be used once while one will not be used at all.

DIRECTIONS: Place the letter next to the disorder in the right-hand column in the blank space next to the pathophysiological condition that matches it most closely. Each letter may be used one time only while some may not be used at all. (5 points)

ORIGINAL VERSION

Match the drugs in Column A with their major desired action in Column B when used as a preoperative medication

Column A	Column B
1. Atropine ____	A. Analgesia
2. Visteral ____	B. Anticholinergic
3. Valium ____	C. Antiemetic
	D. Antianxiety

REVISED VERSION

MATCHING QUESTIONS

DIRECTIONS: Match the drugs in the left-hand column with the major desired action of the drug when used as a preoperative medication which are given in the right-hand column. Each action may be used once, more than once or may not be used at all.

Drugs	Desired Action
(D) 1. Atropine	A. Analgesia
(C) 2. Diazepam (Valium)	B. Antiemetic
(C) 3. Hydroxyzine (Vistaril)	C. Antianxiety
	D. Anticholinergic

Guidelines Violated -- #1, 6, and 7

Both generic and trade names of common drugs should be given. I believe that nurses should know both.

ORIGINAL VERSION

MATCHING - place the letter of your answer from Column A in the spaces provided in Column B. (6 points)

COLUMN A	COLUMN B
A. hemoptysis	____ dram
B. sanguineous	____ after meals
C. tachypnea	____ rapid breathing
D. p.c.	____ bloody sputum
E. orthopnea	____ with
F. ℥	____ right eye
G. o.d.	
H. o.s.	
I. o.v.	
J. ʒ	
K. $\overline{ss}$	
L. $\bar{c}$	

REVISED VERSION

MATCHING QUESTIONS

DIRECTIONS: Match the drug administration terms in the column on the left with the appropriate symbol from the right column. Place the letter in the appropriate space. Each letter is to be used only once while some letters will not be used at all.

Terms	Symbols
(H) 1. dram	A. o.d.
(G) 2. after meals	B. o.s.
(D) 3. with	C. o.v.
(A) 4. right eye	D. $\bar{c}$
	E. $\overline{ss}$
	F. a.c.
	G. p.c.
	H. ʒ
	I. ℥

Guidelines Violated -- #1, 2, 3, 5, and 6. I also made the lists more homogeneous.

ORIGINAL VERSION

DIRECTIONS; Match each of the types of medication orders in Column A with the appropriate definition in Column B. Each of the definitions may be used once, more than once, or not at all.

Column A	Column B
1. ___ PRN order	A. Drug given only once & immediately
2. ___ Single order	B. Drug given only once at the earliest convenient time or at a specified time
3. ___ Stat order	C. Drug given only once when in the nurse's judgement the client needs it
4. ___ Standing order with termination date	D. Drug given for stated number of days or times as ordered
	E. Drug given until discontinued by physician's order

REVISED VERSION

DIRECTIONS: For each of the medication orders in the column on the left, select the correct definition in the right column and insert the corresponding letter in the blank space. Each of the definitions may be used once or not at all.

Medication Orders	Definitions
(C) 1. PRN order	A. Drug given only once and immediately
(A) 2. Stat order	B. Drug given only once at the earliest convenient time or at a specified time
(B) 3. Single order	C. Drug given only once when in the nurse's judgement the client needs it
(D) 4. Standing order with termination date	D. Drug given for stated number of days or times as ordered
	E. Drug given until discontinued by physician's order

Guideline Violated -- #1
NOTE: This set could have had the columns reversed with the student matching the medication orders to the definitions.

ORIGINAL VERSION

Match the hypertensive drug in Column A with its major antihypertensive action in Column B.

Column A	Column B
1. Propranolol___	A. Diuretic
2. Guanethidine___	B. Vasodilator
	C. Post ganglionic sympathetic blocking agent
	D. Beta adrenergic blocking agent

REVISED VERSION

MATCHING QUESTIONS

DIRECTIONS: Match the antihypertensive drug listed in the left-hand column with its major antihypertensive action listed in the right-hand column.Each action may only be used once while one will not be used at all.

Drugs	Actions
(C) 1. Propranolol (Inderal)	A. Sympathetic nervous system inhibitor
(B) 2. Guanethidine (Ismelin)	B. Norepinephrine blocking agent
	C. Beta adrenergic receptor antagonist

Guidelines Violated -- #1 and 6

I added the generic drug names. I also changed the choices in Column B, Actions, to coincide with the literature for content validity.

ORIGINAL VERSION

MATCHING QUESTIONS

Directions: For each of the terms in Column A, match the appropriate description from Column B. Each description in Column B may be used once, more than once or not at all.

Column A	Column B
1. ____ Apnea	A. Cessation of breathing
2. ____ Bradypnea	B. Difficult breathing
3. ____ Dyspnea	C. Increased depth of respiration
4. ____ Eupnea	D. Noisy breathing
5. ____ Hyperpnea	E. Normal, easy breathing
6. ____ Tachypnea	F. Respiratory rate lower than 10 per minute
	G. Respiratory rate over 24 per minute

REVISED VERSION

DIRECTIONS: For each of the respiratory terms in the left-hand column, match the correct description pertaining to respirations from the right-hand column and insert the corresponding letter in the blank space. Each description may be used once, more than once, or not at all.

Terms	Descriptions
(C) 1. Apnea	A. Noisy breathing
(F) 2. Bradypnea	B. Difficult breathing
(B) 3. Dyspnea	C. Cessation of breathing
(D) 4. Eupnea	D. Normal, easy breathing
(E) 5. Hyperpnea	E. Increased depth of respiration
(G) 6. Tachypnea	F. Respiratory rate lower than 10 per minute
	G. Respiratory rate over 24 per minute

Guideline Violated -- #1

ORIGINAL VERSION

Match the following vital signs in the left hand column to the correct term in the right hand column by placing A or B on your answer sheet.

___	B/P 134/86	P 130	T 100^{8}		A. Normal
___	B/P 160/96	P 88	R 36		B. Abnormal
___	B/P 110/68	P81	R 14		

REVISED VERSION

MATCHING QUESTIONS

DIRECTIONS: For each of the sets of vital signs (from adult clients) in the left-hand column, indicate whether it is Normal or Abnormal by placing an A or B in the space next to the appropriate set of vital signs. The letters in the right-hand column may be used once, more than once, or not at all.

Vital Signs					Interpretation
(B) 1.	B/P $\frac{134}{86}$	P 130	T 100^{8}		A. Normal
					B. Abnormal
(B) 2.	B/P $\frac{160}{96}$	P 88	R 36		
(A) 3.	B/P $\frac{110}{68}$	P 81	R 14		

Guidelines Violated -- #1, 6, and 7

ORIGINAL VERSION

MATCHING

Column A	Column B
____ 1. Inflammation of artery	A. Atherosclerosis
____ 2. Plaque formation in artery	B. Coarctation of aorta
____ 3. Arterial stenosis	C. Coronary arteritis

REVISED VERSION

MATCHING QUESTIONS

DIRECTIONS: Place the letter next to the disorder in the right-hand column in the blank space next to the pathophysiological condition that matches it most closely. Each letter may be used once, more than once, or not at all.

Pathophysiology	Disorder
(A) 1. Inflammation of the artery	A. Coronary arteritis
(D) 2. Plaque formation in the artery	B. Coarctation of the aorta
(B) 3. Stricture of the artery	C. Atherosclerosis
	D. Arteriosclerosis

Guidelines Violated -- #1, 4, and 6
I added the word "the" to several of the choices. I believe it enhances readability.

ORIGINAL VERSION

Matching - Place the letter of your answer from Column A in the spaces provided in Column B. (4 points)

Column A	Column B
A. Nursing order	___anger due to diagnosis of fatal disease
B. Deadlines	___verbalization of acceptance of dx
C. Nursing Diagnosis	___time of discharge from hospital
D. Expected outcome	___active listening am and pm shift for 15-20 mins.

REVISED VERSION

MATCHING QUESTIONS

DIRECTIONS: Match the term in the column on the right with the appropriate example in the column on the left and insert the corresponding letter in the blank space. Each letter may be used once while one will not be used at all. (4 points)

Examples	Terms
(B) 1. Anger due to diagnosis of fatal illness	A. Deadlines
(C) 2. Verbalization of acceptance of diagnosis	B. Expected outcome
(A) 3. Time of discharge from hospital	C. Nursing diagnosis
(D) 4. Active listening a.m. and p.m. shifts for 15-20 minutes	D. Nursing order
	E. Physician's order

Guidelines Violated -- #1, 3, 4, and 6

ORIGINAL VERSION

Match the conditions found in surgical clients undergoing general anesthesia in Column A with the nursing conclusions in Column B

Column A	Column B
1. Post-op day 1 Mr. Jones complains of sore throat___	A. Expected post-op response and continue to monitor
2. Cool, pale skin immediately upon arrival from recovery room. Heart rate 105. Urine output 40 cc for last hour___	B. Abnormal response and should be reported to M.D. promptly
3. Post-op day 7 Mr. Jones complains of tender area in left calf area with discomfort noted on sharp dorsiflexion of the left foot___	C. Normal condition and thus no action is needed at this time

REVISED VERSION

MATCHING QUESTIONS

DIRECTIONS: Match the conditions found in surgical clients who have had general anesthesia in the left-hand column with the nursing conclusions in the right-hand column. Insert the appropriate letter in the blank space on the left. Each letter may be used once, more than once, or not at all.

Postoperative Conditions	Nursing Conclusions
(B) 1. Immediately upon arrival from recovery room skin is cool and pale, heart rate is 90, and urine output was 40 cc for last hour	A. Normal condition and therefore no action is needed at this time
(A) 2. Post-op day 1; Mr. Jones complains of a sore throat	B. Expected post-op response but continue to monitor
(C) 3. Post-op day 7; Mr. Jones complains of tender area in left calf. Discomfort noted on sharp dorsiflexion of the left foot	C. Abnormal response and should be reported to the physician promptly
	D. Unexpected but not a serious response; therefore, continue to observe

Guidelines Violated -- #1, 4, 5, and 6

ORIGINAL VERSION

DIRECTIONS: Column A contains a list of signs and symptoms of pregnancy. On the line at the left of each statement put the letter of the category in Column B that best fits the statement. Each response in Column B may be used once or more than once.

Column A	Column B
____ 1. Chadwick's sign	a. Presumptive
____ 2. Fetal heart tones	b. Probable
____ 3. Quickening	c. Positive
____ 4. Uterine souffle	
____ 5. Urinary frequency	

REVISED VERSION

DIRECTIONS: Match the category of signs and symptoms of pregnancy in the right-hand column with the signs and symptoms of pregnancy listed in the left-hand column. Insert the corresponding letter in the blank space. Each response may be used more than once.

Signs and Symptoms of Pregnancy	Category
(C) 1. Chadwick's sign	A. Positive
(A) 2. Fetal heart tones	B. Presumptive
(B) 3. Quickening	C. Probable
(B) 4. Urinary frequency	
(C) 5. Uterine souffle	

Guidelines Violated -- #1 and 5

ORIGINAL VERSION

Under each of the deceleration patterns listed below, list the letter of all appropriate descriptors associated with the deceleration patterns. (3 pts.) Each correct answer is worth 0.25 points. For each incorrect answer 0.25 points will be subtracted.

Early Deceleration

Variable Deceleration

Late Deceleration

A. uniform shape
B. irregular shape
C. synchronous with onset of contraction
D. Depth reflects intensity of contraction
E. Depth variable
F. FHR rarely falls below 110
G. FHR may fall as low as 50
H. Associated with increased FHR baseline
I. Common in late labor
J.

REVISED VERSION

MATCHING QUESTIONS

DIRECTIONS: For each of the deceleration patterns given in the left-hand column, choose ALL of the appropriate descriptors from the right-hand column and insert those letters under the deceleration pattern. Each descriptor may be used once, more than once, or not at all. (13 points)

Deceleration Patterns

Early deceleration

(A, C, D, G, H)

Variable deceleration

(B, E, J, K)

Late deceleration

(A, E, F, I)

Descriptors

A. Uniform shape
B. Irregular shape
C. Synchronous with the onset of contraction
D. FHR rarely falls below 110
E. FHR may fall as low as 50
F. Associated with increased FHR baseline
G. Associated with average baseline
H. Common in late labor
I. Late onset in relation to contraction
J. No relation to onset of contraction
K. Onset and recovery associated with "overshoot"

Guidelines Violated --#1 and 6. Options D and E in the original changed and 2 were added for content validity. The complex scoring was simplified.

ORIGINAL VERSION

All of the following are predisposing factors specific to either placenta previa or abruptio placentae. Please place the appropriate letter by the corresponding descriptive phrase.

A. placenta previa	____ 1. pregnancy-induced hypertension
B. abruptio placentae	____ 2. multiparity
	____ 3. trauma
	____ 4. advanced maternal age
	____ 5. chronic hypertension
	____ 6. vena caval syndrome

REVISED VERSION

MATCHING QUESTIONS

DIRECTIONS: For each of the predisposing factors specific to either placenta previa or abruptio placentae, select the correct condition in the right column and insert the corresponding letter in the blank space. Each of the letters is to be used at least once and may be used more than once.

Predisposing Factors	Conditions
(B) 1. Trauma	A. Placenta previa
(A) 2. Multiparity	B. Abruptio placentae
(A) 3. Multiple pregnancy	
(A) 4. Anatomical anomalies	
(B) 5. Chronic hypertension	
(B) 6. Pregnancy-induced hypertension	

Guidelines Violated -- #1, 3, and 6

Options 4 and 6 in the original changed to 3 and 4 in the revised version for content validity.

ORIGINAL VERSION

Certain orders are commonly associated with the management of a patient hospitalized with a diagnosis of pre-eclampsia. Please match the management procedure with the most appropriate rationale.
(1 pts. each)
(Some choices will not be used at all. Each rationale should be matched with only one management procedure).

A. serial hematocrits
B. force fluids
C. daily weights
D. B/P checks
E. ddaily urine protein checks
F. strict bedrest in a (L) lateral position
C. weekly OCTs

___1. To assess effectiveness of management relative to kidney damage.
___2. To increase the circulating fluid volume.
___3. To detect hemodilution as an index of interstitial fluid mobilization.
___4. To monitor effectiveness of treatment relative to institial fluid mobilization..
___5. To icnrease blood flow to the heart, thereby increasing cardiac output and vital organ profusion.

NOTE: The typographical errors in the stem and options are reproduced as submitted!

REVISED VERSION

MATCHING QUESTIONS

DIRECTIONS: In the right-hand column are some management procedures for a patient with the diagnosis of preeclampsia (pregnancy-induced hypertension). Match the rationale for the procedure given in the left-hand column by placing the most appropriate letter in the blank space. Each letter may only be used once while 2 will not be used at all. (1 point each)

Rationale

(E) 1. To assess the effectiveness of management relative to kidney damage
(B) 2. To monitor fluid balance
(A) 3. To detect hemodilution as an index of interstitial fluid mobilization
(C) 4. To monitor the effectiveness of treatment relative to interstitial fluid mobilization
(F) 5. To increase blood flow to the heart, thereby increasing cardiac output and vital organ perfusion

Procedures

A. Serial hematocrits
B. Intake and output
C. Daily weights
D. Blood pressure checks
E. Daily urine protein checks
F. Strict bedrest in a lateral position
G. Weekly NSTs (non-stress test)

Guidelines Violated --#1, 3, and 7
The phrase "pregnancy-induced hypertension" was added to reflect current terminology and therefore, content validity.

ORIGINAL VERSION

Match the following methods of contraception with the most appropriate descriptive phrase/statement. Some choices may be used more than once, while others may not be used at all.

a, BCP

b. IUD

c. condom

d. diaphram

e. foam

f. jelly/craem

____ Fluctuations in body weight can alter the effectiveness

____ Is/Are thought to decrease the milk production of lactating mothers

____ When used properly can act as both an effective contraceptive agent and deterrent to VD

____ To enhance effectiveness should be used in conjunction with a condom

____ To enhance effectiveness should be used in conjunction with contraceptive jelly/cream

____ An absolute contraindication to use is the presence of acute PID

____ Is/Are the most effective contraceptive agent of those listed

____ Is/Are probably the safest and most effective contraceptive agent of those listed

NOTE: The typographical error and the spelling error are reproduced here as submitted!

REVISED VERSION

MATCHING QUESTIONS

DIRECTIONS: Match the methods of contraception in the right column with the most appropriate description in the left column and insert the corresponding letter in the blank space. Some letters may be used more than once while others may not be used at all. (12 points)

Descriptions		Methods of Contraception
(E)	1. Fluctuations in body weight can alter their effectiveness	A. BCP
(A)	2. Thought to decrease the mile production of lactating mothers	B. IUD
(C,D,F)	3. When used properly, can act as both an effective contraceptive and as a deterrent to VD	C. Foam
(C)	4. Should be used in conjunction with a condom to enhance effectiveness	D. Condom
(D,E)	5. Should be used in conjunction with a contraceptive jelly or cream	E. Diaphragm
(B)	6. An absolute contraindication to use is the presence of acute PID	F. Jelly or cream
(A)	7. The most effective contraceptive agent of those listed	
(E,F)	8. Probably the safest and most effective contraceptive agent of those listed	

Guidelines Violated -- #1, 7, and 8

I reworded some of the descriptions for clarity and to avoid clues. Do not use Is/Are format!

ORIGINAL VERSION

Match the following communicable disease to the appropriate signs. Each letter may be used once, more than once, or not at all.

A. Lesion is marked by patches of grayish membrane
B. Skin eruption which leaves a granular rash
C. Koplik spots on buccal mucosa
D. Diffuse punctate and macular rash
E. Tenderness of salivary and parotid glands

1. Rubella
2. Rubeola
3. Roseola
4. Diphtheria
5. Herpes zoster
6. Mumps

REVISED VERSION

MATCHING QUESTIONS

DIRECTIONS: Place the letter next to the communicable disease in the right-hand column in the blank space next to the sign(s) that matches it most closely. Each letter may be used once, more than once, or not at all.

Signs	Communicable Disease
__(C)__ 1. Koplik spots on buccal mucosa.	A. Mumps
__(D)__ 2. Diffuse maculopapular rash.	B. Rubella
__(A)__ 3. Tenderness of salivary and parotid glands.	C. Rubeola
__(B)__ 4. Skin eruption which leaves a branny rash.	D. Roseola
__(E)__ 5. Lesion is marked by patches of grayish membrane.	E. Diphtheria
	F. Herpes zoster

Guidelines Violated -- #1, 3, and 7. The wording in options B and D was changed to reflect the literature.

GUIDES FOR WRITING COMPLETION QUESTIONS

1. Write the statement in a manner that clearly demands a specific answer.
2. Do not mutilate statements by leaving out too many words. Omit only key words.
3. If specific units or measures are needed, include them in the question, unless of course they are the answer.
4. Whenever possible, the omitted word or words should be at the end of the statement. This practice helps the student to know what is expected. It does ease reading.
5. Be careful about providing unintended cues by grammatical construction.
6. If there is more than one correct answer, the answer key should indicate all acceptable responses.
7. All blanks should be the same length in order to avoid unintended clues.
8. For short answer questions, the same general principles apply except that in this instance you may ask a question.
9. As with other kinds of questions, do not test trivia.
10. Textbook sentences should not be copied with the only difference being the omitted word or words. Use your own words.

COMPLETION QUESTIONS

MATERNITY NURSING

Directions: Insert the word or words that best completes the statement. (1 point each)

1. Spinals, caudals, and epidurals are examples of (regional) anesthesia.
2. In patients who have had spinal, caudal, or epidural anesthesia, peripheral vasodilation may precipitate the occurrence of (maternal hypotension).
3. In helping to prevent a "spinal headache" following spinal anesthesia, it may be helpful to keep the patient in (supine) position for a period of time.
4. The perineum derives its nerve supply primarily from various branches of the (pudendal) nerve.
5. Prompt uterine relaxation is produced by halothane, a (general inhalation) anesthetic agent.
6. When deladumone OB is used, it should be administered at the end of the (second) stage of labor.

SHORT ANSWER AND COMPLETION QUESTIONS--MATERNITY NURSING

DIRECTIONS: For each test question, insert your choices in the appropriate spaces.

1. List 3 indications for terminating a pregnancy complicated by preeclampsia. (3 points)
   1. (Patient becomes eclamptic)
   2. (Patient becomes oliguric/anuric)
   3. (Patient's blood pressure is uncontrollable with the risk of a CVA)
   4. (Patient develops abruptio placentae)
   5. (Patient develops pulmonary edema)
2. Two capabilities of internal mode electronic fetal monitoring NOT achievable by external mode fetal monitoring are: (2 points)
   1. (Can quantify in mm of Hg the intensity of uterine contractions)
   2. (Can quantify in mm of Hg the uterine resting tone between contractions)
3. Two major advantages of external mode electronic fetal monitoring as compared to internal mode fetal monitoring are: (2 points)
   1. (Does not require rupture of the membranes--noninvasive)
   2. (Does not require cervical dilatation)
4. The L/S ratio for fetal lung maturity is determined by what procedure? (1 point)
   (amniocentesis)________________.
5. To assess uterine tone in the postpartum client, the nurse should (1 point) (palpate the fundus)________.

SHORT ANSWER QUESTIONS--VITAL SIGNS

DIRECTIONS: For each test question, insert your choices in the appropriate spaces.

1. List 3 factors that will influence pulse rate.
   1. (Age, size or sex)
   2. (Metabolic rate or drugs)
   3. (Pain or emotions)

2. List 2 events (occurring within ½ hour of the procedure) which may alter an oral temperature.
   1. (Drinking hot or cold fluids)
   2. (Smoking)
      (Chewing gum)

3. List 3 conditions which would make it necessary to take a rectal temperature rather than an oral temperature.
   1. (An unconscious client)
   2. (A disoriented or confused client)
   3. (An infant or young child)
      (Clients having recent rectal surgery)

4. A rectal thermometer is inserted into the adult rectum approximately ______(1½)______ inches.

5. The difference between the systolic and the diastolic pressures is called______(pulse pressure)______.

6. The difference between the apical pulse and the peripheral pulse, if any, is called______(pulse deficit)______.

7. When the pulse rate falls below 50 beats per minute, it is called______(bradycardia)______.

8. When the pulse rate is over 100 beats per minute in an adult client, it is called______(tachycardia)______.

9. If a client's pulse is abnormal in any way, the nurse should count the pulse for a minimum of ______(1 minute)______.

10. The most commonly used site for measuring arterial pulse rates is the ______(radial)______ site.

SHORT ANSWER QUESTIONS - MISCELLANEOUS

Directions: For each test question, insert your choices in the appropriate spaces.

1. List the "Five Rights" of medication administration. (1 point each)
   1. (Right drug)
   2. (Right patient)
   3. (Right time)
   4. (Right route)
   5. (Right amount)

2. List 3 areas that should be assessed for cyanosis in a Black client. (1 point each)
   1. (Buccal mucosa)
   2. (Soles of the feet)
   3. (Palms of the hands)

   (Nail beds)

   (Inferior palpebral conjunctiva)

3. A client's intravenous infusion is not dripping. What 4 steps should be taken to further assess the situation? (1 point each)
   1. (Check for kinked tubing)
   2. (Check to see if the patient is lying on the tubing)
   3. (Observe for infiltration)
   4. (Check to see if the bottle of IV fluid is empty)

   (Check to see if the needle is in the vein)

   (Check to see if blood is in the tubing/needle)

   (Check to see if the tape over the needle is too tight)

FILL-IN QUESTIONS - ASSESSMENT AND MISCELLANEOUS

Directions: Name the physical examination technique that is described by each of the following phrases. (1 point each)

1. (Auscultation)_______ Use of the sense of hearing such as in listening with a stethoscope
2. (Inspection)_______ Use of the eyes to observe
3. (Palpation)_______ Use of the sense of touch to feel or press on the body
4. (Percussion)_______ Use of the fingertips or a rubber hammer to strike or tap a part of the body

Directions: Insert the word or words that best completes the statement. (1 point each)

5. In assessing for cyanosis, the nurse should observe the patient's lips, lower eyelids, mucous membranes, ear lobes, and (nail beds)_______.
6. The QRS interval or complex on a rhythm strip is a graphic recording of the electrical activity generated during (ventricular contraction)____.
7. According to the standards of the American Heart Association, the initial drug which the nurse should administer in cardiac arrest is (sodium bicarbonate)______.
8. A two-and-a-half-year old child should have a total of (20)_________ deciduous teeth.

TRUE/FALSE QUESTIONS

Many instructors fail to use true and false test items because they are of the opinion that such items don't test very much and even if they do, the student has a 50 percent chance of guessing the answer correctly. With a little creativity and the requisite time to construct such items, they can be designed to get at the higher levels of cognition while at the same time reducing the high chance of guessing.

True/false questions can employ various stimuli--certainly written, but also aural recordings such as heart sounds--graphs, tables, patient's charts (facsimiles will do), laboratory reports and the like. Generally, by using such stimuli, the cognitive level required to get the answer right exceeds that of the typical true/false question. Other ways of increasing the difficulty of the item include having the student underline the word or phrase responsible for making the item false and in some instances, you may want the student to correct the statement to make it true. The use of such techniques greatly reduces the chances of students getting the answers right purely by chance. One other method of presenting true/false items, although it does nothing to alter the possibility of getting it right by chance, is to group them under a covering statement or question. It simply is a different method of presenting such questions. One such example follows.

Which of the following characteristics are normal in newborn infants?

____ 1. Mongolian spots

____ 2. Stepping reflex

____ 3. Dancing reflex

____ 4. Crossed eyes

____ 5. Respiratory irregularities

____ 6. Distended abdomen

HELPFUL HINTS FOR WRITING TRUE/FALSE ITEMS

1. Use the true/false format when it is appropriate to do so. It is inappropriate for getting at the level of synthesis but is certainly appropriate for the lower levels of cognition. It is helpful to know which types of items are best for specific objectives.

2. Never, but never, lift statements directly from references for true or false questions. In fact, I can't think of any instances when this practice is permissible. The only thing being tested if you use direct quotes is memory. (There are times, however, when you may use an author's quote to test the student's interpretation of the quote.) The best practice is to use your own words and keep the reading level easy. Use simple words whenever possible. You want the test to assess nursing knowledge, not vocabulary!

3. Try to keep your statements short--both true and false. Generally, it requires more words and qualifications to tell the truth so the true statements tend to be longer. This can be a clue to the test-wise student.

4. In wording your statement, make sure that it is either right or wrong, not partially wrong or partially right. If the difference in rightness or wrongness hangs on one word, I think it unjust. Suppose the student skims over that word or is distracted at that point. I also believe that students are prone to call such questions tricky and I'm inclined to agree with them!

5. Do not include two distinct ideas in one test question. It's better to write two questions. One reason for not pairing up two ideas is that if the student gets it wrong, you won't know if the student lacked the knowledge required to answer both parts or if he or she had half of the necessary knowledge.

6. As with all questions in a test, they should assess important points, not trivia! Since any test is only a sample of the universe of content in a given subject, all of the questions should contribute to the assessment. It is a fact that it is easier to write items testing such points as facts, terms, definitions and the like. It is therefore, not surprising that one sees many items in a test that assess these lower cognitive levels. Try to write questions at the application and analysis levels.

7. Try to avoid negatively worded questions, whether true/false or multiple choice. Answering such questions involves two steps--first the student must answer it positively to himself before he or she can respond to the negative statement. By all means, avoid double negatives, not only in your test questions, but in your writings as well.

8. When stating opinions in the stems of questions, make sure that you cite the source of the opinion--your own or someone else--and be specific. An example--"According to Gerald Caplan,..."

9. It is wise to avoid the use of vague words such as generally, frequently, occasionally since they are usually ambiguous. What frequently means to me may be far from what it means to the examinee. In addition, such words tend to be used in true statements which then may clue the test-wise student.

10. Specific determiners such as Always, Never, All and No tend also to be clues or cues to false statements. Very few things are always true or never done!

11. As with other kinds of questions, try them out on a peer before you administer them to students. It will help to get out any bugs that you've inadvertently built in to the question. You know what you meant but you may not have communicated it as you intended.

GUIDES FOR WRITING TRUE/FALSE QUESTIONS

1. Present only one idea per question, either completely true or completely false. It is not a wise practice to include two ideas, particularly if one idea is true and the other is false.
2. Avoid at all costs complex statements since they tend to test only one's ability to comprehend the written word.
3. Try to avoid writing negative statements because students tend to overlook negative words. As with other kinds of questions, try to state or word them positively.
4. Specific determiners such as all or none tend to be cues to false statements while usually, generally and some tend to be cues to true statements. Therefore, use such qualifying terms with extreme caution.
5. True statements tend to be longer because of the need to qualify the statement. Therefore, avoid clues to the correct answer by length. Try to have them shorter some of the time and longer at other times.

SAMPLE DIRECTIONS FOR TRUE/FALSE QUESTIONS

It is very easy to confuse a handwritten t and f. It is therefore recommended that the student not be required to write either a t or an f. The better practice is to have them either circle the TRUE or FALSE or underline their choice. Since many institutions provide machine-scoring for answer sheets, the practice regarding alternate-response items such as true/false is to have the students blacken or mark the A or 1 (depending on the type of answer sheet used) for the TRUE responses and the B or 2 for the FALSE responses. Your directions to the students should reflect the practice in your school.

Samples

DIRECTIONS: Circle the TRUE if the characteristic is normally present in newborn infants and circle the FALSE if it is not normal.

DIRECTIONS: For each of the following questions, decide whether the statement is true or false. Circle the TRUE for a true statement or FALSE for a false statement.

DIRECTIONS: For each of the following statements, decide if it is true or false. If it is a TRUE statement, mark your answer sheet A; if it is a FALSE statement, mark your answer sheet B.

DIRECTIONS: For each of the following items, decide whether the statement is true or false. Mark your answer sheet (T) for a true statement or (F) for a false statement like this;

T (F)

SAMPLE TRUE/FALSE QUESTIONS--NEWBORN INFANTS

ORIGINAL VERSION

True/False
The following are normal characteristics of the newborn;

____ a. milia
____ b. cephalohematoma
____ c. caput succedaneum
____ d. acrocyanosis
____ e. Hct $\leq$ 40%

REVISED VERSION

True/False Questions

DIRECTIONS: Circle the TRUE if the characteristic is normally present in newborn infants and circle the FALSE if it is not normal.

(TRUE)	FALSE	1. Milia
TRUE	(FALSE)	2. Cephalohematoma
(TRUE)	FALSE	3. Caput succedaneum
(TRUE)	FALSE	4. Acrocyanosis
TRUE	(FALSE)	5. Hct $\leq$ 40%

Comments

The original version is not stated in a manner that clearly identifies the task for the student. It tells you that the characteristics are normal rather than asks you which ones are. The directions and format clarify the task.

SAMPLE TRUE/FALSE QUESTIONS
FUNDAMENTALS OF NURSING

True/False Questions

DIRECTIONS: For each of the following statements, decide if it is true or false. If it is TRUE, mark your answer sheet 1; if it is a FALSE statement, mark your answer sheet 2.

1. Clients confined to bed should have their legs massaged for 3 to 5 minutes each day to help prevent venous stasis.
2. When making an unoccupied bed, the bottom sheet can be tightened securely if pulled on the diagonal and tucked smoothly.
3. Soap is effective because it increases the surface tension of water and acts as an emulsifying agent.
4. Dentures should be cleaned with hot water as this provides for more effective removal of bacterial plaque.
5. When shaving a male patient, the razor should be pulled against the growth of beard.
6. It is not necessary to wash under the foreskin when giving perineal care to an uncircumcised male.
7. Hot water should be used for the initial rinsing of a bed-pan because it dissolves feces.
8. Carbohydrates are generally the main source of energy in the diet.
9. Somnambulism is another name for insomnia.
10. Before taking a temperature with a glass thermometer, the nurse should rinse the chemical solution from the thermometer and then wipe it with a tissue from the bulb toward the finger.
11. The amount of pain experienced is not necessarily in proportion to the amount of damage occurring in the body.

12. Pain may be defined as the sensation of physical and/or mental suffering or hurt that usually causes distress or agony to the one experiencing it.

13. When preparing and administering oral medications, the nurse should use medical asepsis.

14. To make removal of a medication from an ampule easier, the nurse should inject an amount of air equal to the amount of solution to be withdrawn.

15. Medications should be instilled into the eye by applying the solution or ointment directly onto the eyeball.

ANSWERS

1. False	6. False	11. True
2. True	7. False	12. True
3. False	8. True	13. True
4. True	9. False	14. True
5. True	10. False	15. False

SAMPLE TRUE/FALSE QUESTIONS

MISCELLANEOUS

True/False Questions

DIRECTIONS:For each of the following statements, decide if it is true or false. If it is TRUE, mark your answer sheet 1; if it is a FALSE statement, mark your answer sheet 2.

1. In doing a respiratory assessment, instruct the patient to breathe orally and slightly deeper than normal as it increases the intensity of breath sounds.
2. Women normally have diaphragmatic breathing as evidenced by abdominal bulging.
3. Rales and rhonchi should not signify any underlying pathology since they are common findings in adult clients.
4. Of the axillary lymph nodes, the subscapular (posterior) nodes are most often palpable.
5. Most of the tuberculosis seen in adults is of the secondary or reactivated type.
6. Clients on steroids or immunosuppresive therapy have a higher incidence of tuberculosis.

ANSWERS

1. True
2. False
3. False
4. False
5. True
6. True

SAMPLE TRUE/FALSE QUESTIONS

MISCELLANEOUS

True/False Questions

DIRECTIONS: For each of the following statements, decide if it is true or false. If it is a TRUE statement, mark your answer sheet A; if it is a FALSE statement, mark your answer sheet B.

1. Tinkling sounds auscultated below the umbilicus indicate that air is leaking from the stomach into the peritoneal space.

2. When examining the abdomen, auscultation should be done before palpation and percussion.

3. Moist, crackling sounds auscultated in the lung bases indicate that wheezes are present.

4. When assessing breath sounds, the stethescope should be placed in one or two locations on the chest wall.

5. To prevent transmission of an infection, only one stage of the infection-disease cycle needs to be prevented.

6. Infection-control officers are required by the JCAH (Joint Commission on Accreditation of Hospitals) in all hospitals of 200 or more beds.

7. Intake and output measurements are the most accurate indicators of fluid balance.

8. A specific gravity of 1.003 reported on a urine specimen would be expected in a dehydrated patient who is to receive IV therapy.

9. It is an acceptable procedure to place the Foley drainage bag on the stretcher near the patient's leg when transporting him.

10. In turning a patient to a side-lying position, the nurse should place one foot forward to assure a wide base of support, keeping the knees in a locked position.

11. In doing ROM exercises, adduction is defined as moving the arm away from the body.

12. In selecting the ventral gluteal site for an IM injection, the landmarks should be the greater trochanter of the femur, the anterior superior iliac spine, and the iliac crest.

13. The face is customarily washed last when giving a bed bath.

14. A pulse rate of 85 in an adult is classified as tachycardia.

15. An EKG is a diagnostic procedure that measures electrical activity of the brain.

16. Atherosclerosis is the loss of the muscular function within the wall of the artery with subsequent hardening or calcification.

17. The behavior of a patient with a diagnosis of organic brain syndrome is usually passive and predictable.

18. According to Eric Erikson, the infant operates in the stage known as "Trust vs Mistrust".

ANSWERS

1. False	10. False
2. True	11. False
3. False	12. False
4. False	13. False
5. False	14. False
6. False	15. False
7. False	16. False
8. False	17. False
9. False	18. True

SAMPLE TRUE/FALSE QUESTIONS

PREGNANCY

True/False Questions

DIRECTIONS: For each of the following questions, decide whether the statement is true or false. Circle the TRUE for a true statement or FALSE for a false statement.

TRUE (FALSE) 1. The dyspnea of pregnancy is a clinical sign of the increased O_2 utilization of the fetus and mother.

(TRUE) FALSE 2. The RBC mass increases in proportion to the total body fluid volume during pregnancy.

TRUE (FALSE) 3. Pruritis gravidarum occurs because of the increased production of melanin during pregnancy.

(TRUE) FALSE 4. Relaxation of the smooth musculature during pregnancy is due to the effects of estrogen.

TRUE (FALSE) 5. There is a normal increase in the blood pressure of the pregnant woman from the beginning of the second trimester to term.

TRUE (FALSE) 6. Oral hypoglycemics are prescribed for use by a Class B diabetic during pregnancy.

TRUE (FALSE) 7. A woman in the transition phase of labor states that she needs to have a bowel movement. The appropriate nursing action is to place her on a bedpan.

TRUE (FALSE) 8. Pregnancy is diabetogenic because the pregnant woman has a decreased ability to produce insulin.

TRUE (FALSE) 9. The IDM (infant of a diabetic mother) may become hypocalcemic in the nursery because of his immature liver with the resultant inability to conjugate bilirubin.

SAMPLE TRUE/FALSE QUESTIONS

(MATERNITY NURSING)

True/False Questions

DIRECTIONS: For each of the following questions, decide whether the statement is true or false. Circle the TRUE for a true statement or FALSE for a false statement.

TRUE (FALSE) 1. The greater immaturity of the sympathetic nervous system as compared to the parasympathetic nervous system of the fetus may account for the occurrence of more decelerations than accelerations.

TRUE (FALSE) 2. Bradycardia may be an early sign of fetal distress.

(TRUE) FALSE 3. One pathological mechanism contributing to placental insufficiency in a class F diabetic woman is reduced placental growth.

ESSAY QUESTIONS

Essay questions, like other kinds of paper-and-pencil questions, have been misused, abused, overused, and underused in examinations. They can be designed, however, to serve many specific purposes. The information that can be obtained from well-designed essay questions is not obtainable from other objective paper-and-pencil measures. The following section will provide information about the advantages of essay questions, some guidelines for developing them, and finally some hints for scoring essay questions as objectively and fairly as possible.

Major Advantages of Essay Questions

1. The assessment of knowledge at the level of synthesis is probably the chief advantage of essay questions. Inherent in the task of synthesizing knowledge is the need to create, design or construct something whole and new from the parts. This task cannot be accomplished by providing students with choices such as in a multiple-choice question. Since one or more of our objectives in the health professions should be aimed at this level of cognition, I would hope that somewhere in our evaluation procedures there is a place for essay questions.

2. Another major advantage of essay questions is their ability to assess problem-solving and decision-making skills of students. Inherent in such skills is the need to organize and integrate knowledge as a prerequisite to the application of such knowledge. In order to create a novel or new approach to a specified problem, the student must garner all of the facts, principles and concepts at his command in order to design his or her answer. If we in the health professions truly want our graduates to be innovative and creative in approaches to client care, then we need to provide them with opportunities to demonstrate such abilities.

Types of Essay Questions

Basically the two types of essay questions are 1) the extended response and 2) the limited or restricted response. My preference is for the second type because, in general, I don't want students to tell me everything they know about a topic but rather to focus on a particular point and synthesize knowledge to arrive at a solution to the specified problem. In most instances, this can be accomplished in 1 or 2 pages. At the level of education in which we are involved and with the caliber of students with whom we are engaged, they should be able to accomplish this task with relative ease.

With either type of essay question, the structure of the question is extremely important. What we want students to do in responding to the question will be determined by the question's structure. The more the question is structured, the more structured the response will be (and the less disorganized and rambling.)

Guidelines for Writing Essay Questions

1. Examine your course, unit and class objectives to see which ones must be or can best be evaluated by essay questions. Objectives that begin with the verb "Synthesize" are obvious candidates for essay questions. Since essay questions should be reserved for assessing the more complex objectives, other verbs that will provide clues are "Critique," "Analyze," "Evaluate," "Compare," "Contrast," "Defend," "Predict," "Differentiate," and "Illustrate."

2. The use of a test blueprint or table of specifications will also provide information about the content and/ or objectives that should or could be evaluated by essay questions.

3. Write the question in such a way as to make clear exactly what is wanted in the answer. As with other questions, avoid ambiguous wording. The amount of detail and the expected depth of response should be specified. One way of

indicating the length of response desired is by the amount of space allocated for the question. Another way is by stating "In 1 or 2 pages...." or "In 1 or 2 paragraphs...." in the question itself.

4. Remember to require a new or novel approach to a problem since we want more than the repetition of facts, either from a textbook or lecture notes.

5. If required to answer the question, present the necessary chart, data, graph, laboratory results, or diagram, preferably on the same page with the question. Such material should not be unnecessarily reduced in size (for ease in reading) and should be a quality reproduction.

6. If the assigned task is to defend a position and to cite specific data to support or refute that position, make the task clear to the students. If the data the student provides supports <u>his</u> position, credit should be awarded regardless of the position he chose.

7. Present the same questions to all students. Do not give them a choice of questions to answer, e.g., " Choose three of the five essay questions...." By allowing students such a choice, you are essentially giving different exams to the students and have no basis for the comparison of scores. In addition, by presenting the same questions to all students, you are conveying the intent that the questions are directly related to the objectives. The same practice applies to the use of optional questions, namely, there will be no way of making comparisons.

<u>Directions to the Students for Answering the Essay Questions</u>

At the beginning of the section on essay questions, give some general rules or guidelines for answering the questions. Specific directions may be included in each question which will allow tailoring of the directions to that question. For example, the time parameters for one question may be very different from another one. For some questions you may allow students to outline their answers while in others you may want more detail. In addition, the number of points allocated for each question may vary widely. For one question you may award 20 points while for another, you may award 5 or 10 points. In allotting time constraints, remember that you should be more interested in the amount of knowledge the student possesses, not how fast he or she can answer. In other words, we should be more concerned with testing knowledge and the use of knowledge rather than the speed with which one responds.

The weighting of questions and/or parts of a question should be indicated for each one. Along with the time constraints, the student will be able to tell which items are most important and devote more time to those questions, if he so chooses. Additionally, the amount of space allowed for responding should also be an indication of the question's worth. For some questions you wish to state, "In 1 or 2 pages...." while in others you may wish to say, "In the space that follows...." and then leave a third or quarter of a page blank for their response.

In summary, providing the students with the worth of a question in terms of points and the time limits suggested for each question, will allow the student some input into where he or she will devote the majority of his time. In addition, it should eliminate ambiguity regarding the parameters of each item.

Tips for Scoring Essay Questions

1. The most important maxim in scoring essay questions is to have first prepared a model answer. By doing so, it often helps in clarifying the question by pointing out potential ambiguities. Revising or modifying the question will often result in the presentation of a much clearer problem statement.

2. Indicate the number of points to be awarded to each part of the question, if this is appropriate. The result of allocating points to each part will enable the instructor to be more consistent in grading or scoring the answers.

3. Try to avoid knowing who wrote the answer. This will necessitate that students not write their name on each page of the examination which is a common practice.

4. It is also helpful to have the students start each essay question on a new page. It will then be possible to read all of the answers to one question before going on to read all of the students' responses to the second question and so on.

5. Whenever possible, and especially if it is an important examination such as a final comprehensive one, have more than one instructor grade the answers. Following the independent grading, the instructors can then confer to resolve any discrepancies.

6. After grading all of the responses to the first essay question, rearrange the papers. Do the same thing after reading and grading all of the answers to the next question. This practice will help to eliminate any potential bias.

7. Because I believe that we have a hard enough time assessing knowledge in our own field, I don't think credit should be taken away for grammar, misspelled words and punctuation. I believe there are other opportunities to do that. I am not suggesting that such items are not important! I am just saying that we should assess nursing knowledge or medical knowledge, not basic English!

Later on in this section I have provided a number of examples of essay questions, all with a model answer. As you will see, some of the model answers are rather detailed while others are more sketchy. When you design your own answers, it would be wise to include, at a minimum, what you would like your students to include.

CHECKLIST FOR ESSAY QUESTIONS

1. Is the question appropriate and efficient for the essay format? Does the verb require more than recall of information, such as "Explain" rather than "List"?

2. Is each part of the question clearly identified? It will be easier to grade if you separate "Describe and give an example of...."

3. Is the question reflective of one or more course, unit, or class objective?

4. Is the question clear and unambiguous, and does it define the task?

5. Is there an indication of the questions's importance in points awarded for a correct response?

6. Is there an indication of the time allowed for answering the question?

7. Is there an appropriate amount of space allotted for the answer? A brief response will require about one-half a page while there will be times when you will want to tell students to use the reverse side of the paper for an extended response.

8. Does the question pose a new, unfamiliar or novel approach to a problem? A question that requires problem-solving or the creation of a solution is more appropriate for an essay question than one which requires a lower level of cognitive activity.

9. Are the necessary stimuli included? If the question requires the interpretation of data, are the data provided?

10. Have you prepared the answer guide or model answer?

ESSAY QUESTION

Question

Analyze 1 major theory of learning.

Include -

1. at least 1 person related to this theory,
2. the major concepts, and
3. its application to nursing.

TIME - 30 minutes POINTS - 20

Answer

1. Name of theory and theorist	2 points
2. Motivation	5 points
a. Rewards	
b. Stimulus	
3. Behavior	4 points
4. Application	9 points
a. Domains	
b. Examples	

ESSAY QUESTION

Question

Explain fully but succinctly the General Adaptation Syndrome (G.A.S.).

Use the space provided for your response.

TIME - 20 minutes POINTS - 30

Answer

1. Stage of alarm (10 points)
   a. Neuro alert
   b. Endocrine alert
2. Stage of resistance (10 points)
   a. Neuro response
   b. Endocrine response
3. Stage of exhaustion (10 points)
   a. Death
   b. Medical and nursing intervention

ESSAY QUESTION

Question

Predict 2 possible complications of bed rest for each body system.

Give the rationale for each choice.

Explain 2 nursing measures that could be implemented to prevent each complication.

TIME - 30 minutes 40 POINTS

Answer

SCORE - 8 points x 5 systems = 40 points

1. Cardiac
   Thrombosis formation - ↓ circulation - anatomy and physiology, ROM, turning every 2 hours
   Edema of extremities - ↓ circulation - elevate dependent parts, TED hose
2. Respiratory
   Atelectasis - pooling of fluid in lungs - turn, cough and deep breathe every 2 hours
   Pneumonia - pooling of fluid in lungs - turn, cough, and deep breathe every 2 hours
3. G.U.
   Calculi - loss of calcium from bone - ↑ P.O. fluids, ↓ Ca+ intake
   U.T.I. - stasis of urine, ↑ P.O. fluids, cranberry juice
4. Skeletal
   Decubiti - prolonged pressure with ischemia - massage bony prominences, apply lotion, turn every 2 hours
   Deformity (Contractures) - improper alignment, anatomy and physiology - ROM, exercises - proper positioning
5. G.I.
   Constipation - ↓ peristalsis - ↑ pooling of fluid - ↑ roughage
   Stress ulcers - ↑ anxiety leads to ↑ HCL acid - allow client to verbalize, occupational therapy

ESSAY QUESTION

Question | TIME - 10 minutes | POINTS - 10

Identify 5 signs of cardiogenic shock.

Briefly discuss the pathophysiology that produces each of these symptoms.

Answer

Decreased pumping ability of the heart leads to decreased amount of cardiac output which leads to decreased blood flow to vital organs which leads to increase in heart rate as compensatory mechanism

OR

$\downarrow$ pumping ability of the heart $\rightarrow$ $\downarrow$ amount of cardiac output $\rightarrow$ $\downarrow$ blood flow to vital organs $\rightarrow$ $\uparrow$ in heart rate as compensatory mechanism

ESSAY QUESTION

Question TIME - 10 minutes;POINTS- 10

List 3 signs or symptoms that accompany acute pulmonary edema.

Discuss nursing measures specific for each sign or symptom listed.

Answer

1. Dyspnea
   a. Elevate head of bed
   b. Administer oxygen
2. Moist, bubbly rales
   a. Elevate head of bed
   b. Decrease IV rate to keep vein open
3. Anxious
   a. Administer oxygen
   b. Offer reassurance

ESSAY QUESTION -- MATERNITY NURSING

Question

Formulate a theory for the onset of labor.

Include the relevant aspects of anatomy and physiology.

TIME- 20 minutes POINTS - 20

Answer

1. Stretch response of the cervix from the presenting part
   a. Release prostaglandin from the cells of the cervix
   b. Prostaglandin increases receptivity of the uterus to oxytocin
2. Stimulation of the posterior pituitary to release oxytocin
3. Onset of labor because oxytocin stimulates uterine contractions

ESSAY QUESTION -- MATERNITY NURSING

Patient Situation

Mrs. Brennar, 30 years old, is admitted to the labor and delivery suite in active labor at the 37th week of gestation. She is expecting twins.

Essay Question

(TIME- 20 minutes; POINTS - 20)

Identify 3 factors that are contributing to her high-risk status.
Discuss briefly the physiologic significance of each factor.
Indicate how each of the physiologic factors could affect Mrs. Brennar's postpartum psychological adaptation.

Answer

	Physiologic	Psychological
1. Maternal age	↑ risk of Down Syndrome	Generativity vs expanding family
	Prolonged labor	Possible C section
2. Twins	↑ risk intrapartal accidents	↑ tasks for mother ↑ fatigue - sleep deprivation
	↑ risk of prematurity	↑ expense
3. Prematurity	↑ respiratory problems - infant	Separation - bonding
		↑ expense
	Infections	Infant response → bonding ↑ mothering
	Feedings	
		Family dysfunction
4. Surgery	Anesthesia	Recovery postpartum slowed
	Effects of major surgery	Fatigue
		↑ expense

ESSAY QUESTION

(MATERNITY NURSING)

Question

Compare a premature infant and a term (AGA) infant in terms of

a. surface characteristics

b. neurobehavioral characteristics.

Indicate the appropriate parent teaching that should be done prior to discharge and directed toward the

c. physical needs of each infant

d. psychosocial needs of each infant.

You will have 30 minutes to answer this question. It may be done in outline form. (30 points)

Answer

a. Surface Characteristics

Term Infant	Premature Infant
Vernix ↓	Vernix ↑
Little lanugo	↑ lanugo
Ear cartilage	Lack of ear cartilage
Foot creases	↓ foot creases
Subcutaneous fat	Little subcutaneous fat
Breast tissue 7-10 mm	Breast tissue below 4-5 cm
Skin-absence of veins	Skin-translucent
Hair-single strand (NOT WITH BLACKS)	Hair-wooly
Genitalia	Genitalia
Male-full rugae	Male-little rugae
testicles down	undescended testes
Female- labia majora	Female-clitoris prominent
covers clitoris	labia majora small,
	widely separated

b. Neurobehavioral Characteristics

Term Infant	Premature Infant
Square window-turn $\downarrow$ 30° angle	Angle is 90° or more
Sucking-strong	Present at 32 weeks
Sucking and swallowing synchronized	Under 32 weeks, sucking not synchronized with swallow
Cry-lusty and strong	Weak cry
Scarf sign- elbow at midline	Elbow passes midline
Grasp-can lift baby off bed	Weak grasp
Heel to ear- $\uparrow$ resistance	Under 30 weeks, no resistance
Posture- flexion	Hypotonic posture
State behavior- organized	State behavior-unorganized

c. Physical needs of each infant

NEED

Continuity of care upon discharge

Pediatrician identified or Well Baby Clinic-seen at 2-4 weeks of age	Same See at 2 weeks of age

Nutrition

Nurse on demand	Same
Breast-nurses more frequently than bottle fed <u>OR</u>	Same-not pooled but from own mother
Bottle-teach aseptic technique Feed q 3-5 hours	Same Bottle feed q 3 hours and may take longer

For both- Breast or bottle-fed first 4-6 months; raw cow's milk only after 12 months of age

Burping

When the baby needs it	More often than full-term

Bath	
Sponge bath until cord heals (Newly reported-tub baths)	Same Special precautions to prevent cold stress
Safety	
Obtain car seat	Same but will need to pad around baby
Clothing	
Layette	Same but may need extra clothing to prevent cold stress
Taking axillary temperature	
Same	Same
Teaching signs and symptoms of infection	
Same	Same but increased precautions as preterm more at risk
Changing diapers and genital care	
Same	Same but discuss where "premie" diapers may be obtained Discuss how genitals will change with age
Cord care	
Same	Same but cord may be off if had an umbilical catheter
Circumcision care	
Same	Same but may not have been done if a very small infant
Sleep	
Same	Initially will have less awake time
State behavior learning	
Infant stimulation techniques	Less organized Do not overstimulate or understimulate

Brazelton's assessment of behavior

Teach individual characteristics of the baby	Baby less able to organize behavior

d. Psychosocial Needs

Interactional ability and effect on bonding attachment

Milestones related to social behavior	Delay in milestones due to immaturity of CNS

Baby's need to interact with entire family

Same	Same but do not overstimulate

AN ESSAY QUESTION USING DIAGRAMS

1. Identify the cardiac defect represented by each of the 3 diagrams.

   Describe the relevant anatomical and physiological differences from the normal adult heart for each.

   Explain the presence or absence of cyanosis for each.

   (30 minutes; 30 points)

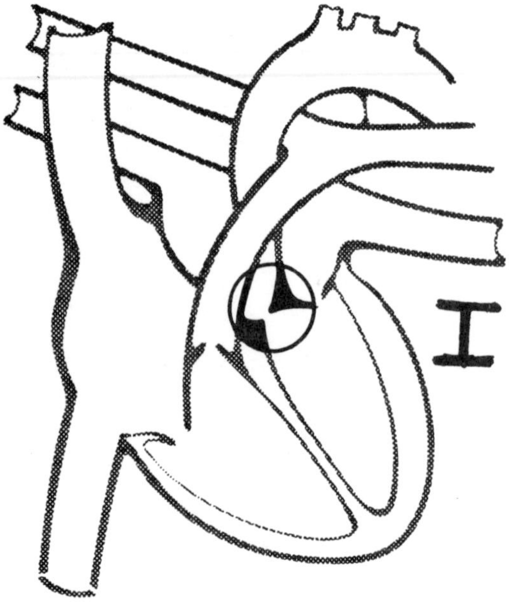

I

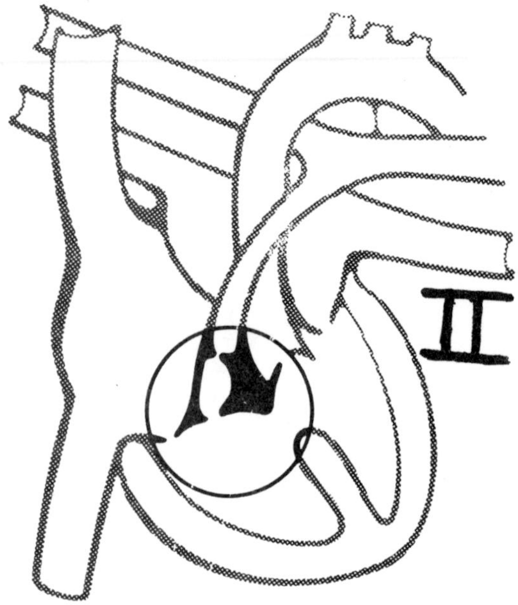

II

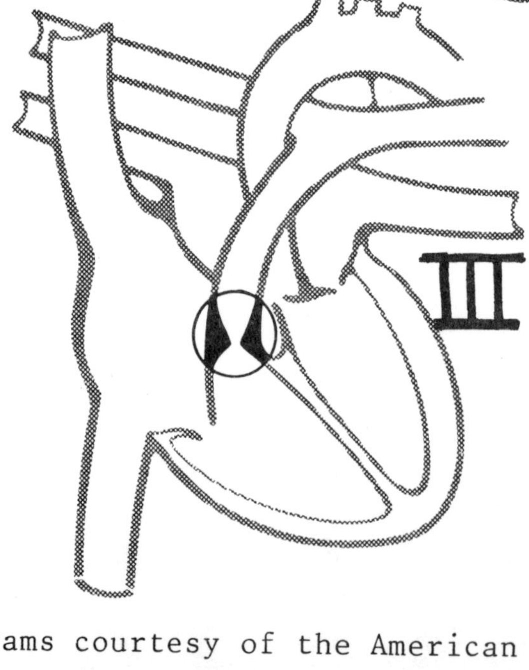

III

NOTE: Diagrams courtesy of the American Heart Association.

SUGGESTED ANSWER TO CARDIAC QUESTION

I. Aortic Stenosis (1 point)

Aortic valve orifice is narrowed impeding the flow of blood from the left ventricle during systole. To pump the blood through the stenotic valve requires increased ventricular pressure. To produce this increased pressure, the left ventricle hypertrophies. (5 points)

The blood is oxygenated and there is not an increased amount of reduced hemoglobin so cyanosis is not a feature of aortic stenosis. (4 points)

II. Tetralogy of Fallot (1 point)

With Tetralogy of Fallot, there is an interventricular septal defect (often large) providing a direct opening between the right and left ventricles. Since the left ventricular pressure is much greater than the right ventricular pressure during systole, blood should be shunted from the left side to the right side but there is also a pulmonic stenosis in Tetralogy. The pulmonic valve orifice is narrowed impeding the blood flow from the right ventricle into the pulmonary arteries during systole. Additionally, the aorta overrides the two ventricles; that is, the aorta is dextrapositioned. This places the aorta at the location of the septal defect. During systole with the pulmonary stenosis, the path of blood exit becomes the aorta for both right and left ventricle content. Hence, a large right-to-left shunt is present. (5 points)

This is the most common pediatric cyanotic heart disease. The degree of pulmonary stenosis determines the amount of deoxygenated blood exiting through the aorta, so the degree of cyanosis is indicative of the degree of shunting and pulmonary stenosis. (4 points)

III. Pulmonary (Tricuspid valve) Stenosis (1 point)

The pulmonic valve orifice is narrowed impeding the flow of blood from the right ventricle during systole. To pump blood through the stenotic valve requires increased ventricular pressure. To produce this increased pressure the right ventricle hypertrophies. (5 points)

The venous blood has increased amounts of reduced hemoglobin because of slowed circulation time from increased venous pressure. There may be <u>some</u> mild cyanosis in severe right ventricular failure but pulmonary stenosis is considered an acyanotic heart disease in children because one doesn't have deoxygenated blood mixing with oxygenated blood. (4 points)

ESSAY QUESTION

Question

Describe Gerald Caplan's Theory of Crisis Intervention.
Explain the phases of crisis.
Formulate therapeutic nursing interventions for each phase.

POINTS - 20 TIME - 30 minutes

Answer

I. 1. Caplan's definition of crisis (2 points)
A crisis is an upset in the individual's steady state. It is a time-limited period of psychological disequilibrium. A sudden change in a life situation which is either internally or externally produced - with which the individual is immediately unable to cope.

2. Common characteristics of crisis (2 points)
Persons in crisis reach out for help and are more vulnerable to the help of others. They are, therefore, more susceptible to help from professionals. They may express the need for help verbally or non-verbally. How one responds to crisis varies depending upon their perception i.e., if one perceives the crisis as a threat, the predominant behavior is anxiety. If one perceives the crisis as a loss (real or imagined), the predominant behavior will be depression. If one perceives the crisis as a challenge his behavior will show some anxiety; however, the ↑ energy from this anxiety is channeled into purposeful problem-solving.

3. Factors influencing (2 points)
   Such factors include: the person's perceptions of the crisis, whether the perception is realistic, how long, how serious and how unexpected was the event precipitating crisis. What are the person's strengths - what coping behaviors has he used in the past that he may be able to call upon now? What is the individual's general state of health? What kind of support systems are available i.e., social, cultural and situational support. Also, does anyone share the crisis.

II. Phases:

Impact (2 points)
The first phase may be characterized by feelings of bewilderment, confusion, disbelief, or denial. Many people experience an <u>unreal</u> feeling about what is happening. This phase may last from a few minutes to a few days.

Turmoil (2 points)
Behaviors common in this phase are anxiety, depression, anger, guilt, withdrawal and any number of somatic complaints. People often feel disorganized, less efficient, tense and often engage in meaningless behaviors.

Resolution (2 points)
In the resolution phases, persons find alternative ways to cope or reduce the anxiety and tension. They begin to mobilize defenses. Resolution is the turning point. The person may become worse and experience further psychological disequilibrium. He may simply return to his previous behavior pattern without experiencing any appreciable change <u>or</u> he may find new ways to cope, learn new things about himself and come out of the crisis a better, stronger person.

III. Nursing interventions (8 points)

First of all, people in crisis are reaching out. Respond to them. Get close to them. Help them face the reality of the situation. Find out how they perceive what is happening to them. Help them view it realistically. It helps to let them know the duration of the crisis and the intensity of the feelings they will experience. Help them to mobilize their support systems if available. Short bursts of intervention are helpful - brief periods of interaction may be most helpful. Focus on the present crisis. It is helpful to decrease anxiety by giving a person <u>something</u> to do. People in crisis may need direction. If anger is expressed - allow it and do not respond defensively. Be empathetic. Allow the person to express and experience what they feel. It is healthy.

ESSAY QUESTION

Question

Discuss the stages of the grief process as described by Kubler-Ross.

Describe 2 nursing interventions for each.

POINTS - 25 TIME - 30 minutes

Answer

1. Denial (1 point)
   A. Don't strip patient of defenses but don't lie to him. Be honest - reality-oriented. (2 points)
   B. Let the patient know you are ready to discuss his feelings, fears and that he won't be abandoned. (2 points)
2. Anger (1 point)
   A. Let the patient express the anger. Do not take it personally. Acknowledge his feelings. (2 points)
   B. Try to remain with the patient so he sees his anger doesn't drive you away. (2 points)
3. Bargaining (1 point)
   A. This stage may go unnoticed but if not, be empathetic. Remember it is helpful to the patient. (2 points)
   B. If the patient discusses these thoughts, be open and allow him to express. (2 points)
4. Depression (1 point)
   A. Allow the patient to mourn, cry and talk about his losses. (2 points)
   B. Recognize that depression is a normal part of grieving and that the person <u>needs</u> to express these feelings freely. (2 points)
5. Acceptance (1 point)
   A. Allow patient to be calm and quiet - detached. Do not force interaction. (2 points)
   B. Remain with the patient and be supportive. (2 points)

ESSAY QUESTION

Question

Describe the pathophysiological changes associated with left ventricular failure so as to account for

A. pressure changes within the heart chambers and pulmonary circulation;
B. signs and symptoms observed in the client;
C. nursing interventions related to the management of signs and symptoms.

TIME - 30 minutes POINTS - 15 1-2 pages

A.	B.	C.
Left ventricular myocardium has decreased contractility → ↓ cardiac output →	sinus tachycardia	Bedrest to ↓ O_2 demand and work of heart Administer prescribed drug therapy to ↑ contractility and slow heart
↓ Impaired left ventricular emptying ↓ Increased left end - diastolic volume and pressure ↓ Impaired left atrial emptying ↓ Increased left atrial volume and pressure ↓ Increased pulmonary venous pressure ↓ Increased capillary pressure → pulmonary edema →	Dyspnea including PND and orthopnea Rales Hemoptysis ↓ PO_2 → hypoxia → anxiety	Positioning Pulmonary hygiene measures: turn, cough, deep breathing exercises Oxygen therapy and support
↓ Increased pulmonary artery pressure ↓ Impaired right ventricular emptying ↓ Increased right end -diastolic volume and pressure ↓ Impaired right atrial emptying ↓ Increased systemic venous pressure → decreased venous return → ↓ Increased capillary pressure →	Cyanosis Hepatomegaly Peripheral edema	Positioning Skin care
	Gut engorgement → anorexia and nausea	Small meals Mouth care
		Fluid restriction and diuresis comes from all aspects of volume expansion

SECTION 3: OTHER DIMENSIONS OF TEST CONSTRUCTION

VALIDATION OF CORRECT ANSWERS

Experience has taught me how important it is to document your correct answer to every question, regardless of format. I also suggest that you negate each of your false choices--that is, make sure that they are absolutely wrong! The process of documenting the correct answer and negating the wrong ones is very time consuming but I think it is a highly desirable thing to do. For one thing, it does prove to you that you do have only one correct answer and for another, it is very helpful when students challenge you about the correctness of a particular item with the possibility that another option may be correct. You can then whip out your test question with the documentation on it and say to the student that Waley and Wong (assume that this is the students' textbook) on page 324 support the correct answer and on pages 322 and 323 negate the other choices. How much easier such a confrontation can be when you have the evidence in front of you!

What I suggest is that, at a minimum, you use the course textbook as your reference. I would supplement that reference with current nursing and medical journals as necessary. We all know how soon textbooks become outdated in our highly complex, technological profession. I am sure that you include such current reference materials on your bibliographies and alert students to material that has just been published. In addition to the references already cited, I also suggest that you use the medical tomes as necessary, particularly for information that is unlikely to be found in the nursing texts--drug actions on a particular body system, comprehensive laboratory results, physiological manifestations and adaptations and the like.

For ease in finding additional information in the future, should you need it, include the author's name, the title of the book, the edition if indicated and of course, the page numbers. For journals, include enough information so that the journal can be easily retrieved.

If in the course of checking out your choices, you discover that one of your intended wrong answers has an element of truth in it, it will need to be revised. There should be only one, repeat one, correct answer. This statement applies whether the question is a single-option multiple-choice, combination-type multiple-choice, true/false, or matching. With completion and essay questions, there may be more than one correct answer though obviously you had one in mind when you wrote it and the way you worded it should help in getting the desired response.

Should you find a discrepancy in the correctness of a particular question, you may wish to revise it or discard it. One way to revise the question is to include the source (the authority) in the question--for example, "According to Reva Rubin,..."

The following example shows partial documentation for a true/false question. It could, of course, also be documented by using other references.

EXAMPLE

1. TRUE FALSE The Dubowitz scale assesses both physical and neurological maturity of the newborn.

Validation for #1

Wieczorek, Rita and Janet Natapoff. A Conceptual Approach to the Nursing of Children: Health Care from Birth Through Adolescence. Philadelphia: J. B. Lippincott Co., 1981.

Pages 183 and 187 support the content as correct.

Behrman, Richard E. and Victor C. Vaughn, III. Nelson Textbook of Pediatrics. 12th ed. Philadelphia: Saunders, 1983.

Pages 343 and 344 support the content as correct.

EXAMPLE OF DIFFERENT LEVELS OF SIMILAR CONTENT

SITUATION:

Mrs. Gertrude Brenner, 30 years old, is admitted to the obstetric unit in active labor at the 37th week of gestation. She is expecting twins. Her pregnancy has been uncomplicated.

1. Upon admission, the initial nursing action should be to

    1. administer a cleansing enema.
    * 2. auscultate the fetal heart rates.
    3. insert a foley catheter.
    4. perform a perineal prep.

2. Mrs. Brenner's membranes rupture spontaneously. Of the following actions, the nurse should first

    * 1. check the fetal heart rates.
    2. examine her for engagement of fetal presenting parts.
    3. take Mrs. Brenner's vital signs.
    4. time Mrs. Brenner's contractions.

3. Which of the following measures should be included in Mrs. Brenner's plan of care?

    1. Administering ordered analgesics as frequently as possible because of the severe pain associated with multiple births.
    2. Inserting a foley catheter because an accurate record of output is essential.
    * 3. Monitering fetal heart tones of both fetuses because anoxia is more likely to occur with multiple births.
    4. Preparing her for a cesarean section because of the expected multiple births.

NOTE: These three questions would obviously not be used in the same test because they all test essentially the same content.

DISCUSSION OF ITEMS ON PREVIOUS PAGE

The first question can be answered on the basis of memory if, in class, the instructor had stated that the first thing to do when a woman is admitted to the hospital in labor is to listen to fetal heart tones and/or time her contractions. However, since timing her contractions is not among the choices, then listening to the fetal heart tones would be the best of those presented. Since the same content is presented in most obstetric nursing books, the same low level of recall may also account for answering the question correctly.

The second question may also be answered by recalling what the instructor presented in class or could be remembered from content presented in the textbook. Since one of the distractors (#4) does involve timing her contractions, the question results in a somewhat higher level because of the need to discriminate the action that has priority.

The third question is likely to be more difficult because each option has both a measure in it as well as a rationale for that measure. It is entirely possible, however, for a student to get credit for answering the question correctly just by knowing what action needs to be taken and not having any idea about the reason for that action. One of the disadvantages of writing questions and/or answers with two or more parts is that the instructor will never know whether students have the necessary knowledge to answer the entire question or if they only had part of the necessary knowledge but got the answer correct anyway. (One way for the instructor to find out if the students have all of the knowledge contained in a particular question is to ask them outright, say in class or conference.) If it is important to know if students have the knowledge contained in both parts of an answer, it would be better to write two separate questions.

One of my reasons for including three sample questions assessing essentially the same content is to show how a number of approaches can be used to get at a particular point. Since I believe that examinations should differ from class to class and year to year, building up a reservoir of test questions will enable you to assemble a different examination whenever the need arises.

It is wise, however, to check old items for face and content validity. The stem of the question may contain information that is outmoded, a treatment that is no longer advocated, a treatment that is of questionable efficacy, or the practice may be obsolete, for example, smallpox vaccinations. In addition, the answer may no longer be correct or one or more of the distractors may now be correct. Be sure to look at the item along with the data--the data may be perfectly acceptable but the item no longer has content validity.

AN EXAMPLE SHOWING THAT MANY APPROACHES CAN BE USED TO TEST ESSENTIALLY THE SAME CONTENT

(Only one should be used in an examination)

I believe that each faculty member (or team responsible for the same subject) should build up a reservoir of test questions. If it is important to test a particular point, it will be necessary to have a variety of questions to assess that point. In so doing, a different question can be used each semester for a period of two or three years. Questions can then be recycled if the content is still current and appropriate and if item analysis data are satisfactory.

Miss Diane Dawson, a 58-year-old cashier, is admitted to the hospital with an acute exacerbation of chronic obstructive pulmonary emphysema.

A. In caring for Miss Dawson, it is essential for the nurse to understand that

1. high levels of oxygen stimulate the carotid receptors.
* 2. high levels of oxygen depress the respiraory center.
3. carbon dioxide can depress the respiratory center when it is present in large quantities.
4. carbon dioxide depletion is common in clients with respiratory disease.

B. The nurse assesses Miss Dawson and detects an increased respiratory rate of 42 per minute and cyanosis. Miss Dawson, who is in bed, is also apprehensive. The first actions by the nurse should be to

1. position her on her side and offer her oxygen.
* 2. position her in high-Fowler's and administer oxygen at 2 liters per minute.
3. position her in semi-Fowler's and administer oxygen at 4 liters per minute until her nail-beds are pink.
4. position her for comfort and administer oxygen at 5 liters per minute.

The results of Miss Dawson's arterial blood gases follow:

pH 7.33: pO_2 36:; pCO_2 66.

(Normal blood gas values are: pH 7.35 - 7.45; pO_2 80 - 100; pCO_2 35 - 45 mm/Hg.)

C. All of the following actions are appropriate. Which pair should be taken first?

1. Assess the patient and prepare for emergency interventions.
2. Redraw blood for arterial gases and start oxygen at 35% by mask.
* 3. Have the physician notified immediately and assess the patient.
4. Have the physician notified immediately and prepare the patient for transfer to the Intensive Care Unit.

Miss Dawson's arterial blood gases on admission follow:

pH 7.3; pO_2 50; pCO_2 60.

D. Which of the following physician's orders should the nurse <u>question</u>?

1. IPPB with normal saline q.i.d.
2. Postural drainage with cupping t.i.d.
* 3. Oxygen per nasal cannula at 8 liters per minute.
4. 1,000 cc 5% dextrose in water with Aminophyllin 500 mg at 75 cc per hour.

E. The admitting nurse notes that Miss Dawson is lethargic and irritable, and her color is dusky. She is tachypneic with her respirations at 42 per minute. Which of these nursing interventions would be most appropriate?

1. Restrict her fluid intake.
2. Keep her awake.
3. Place her in reverse Trendelenburg position.
* 4. Give her oxygen at 2 liters per minute by nasal cannula.

F. Miss Dawson's admission orders include the following; "Oxygen at 2 liters per minute." The rationale for a low oxygen flow rate is Miss Dawson's

1. acidosis.
2. hypocarbia.
* 3. hypoxic drive.
4. chronic anemia.

G. What would you expect Miss Dawson's initial arterial blood gases to show?

1. Increased pH and pCO_2 and decreased pO_2.
2. Increased pH and pO_2 and decreased pCO_2.
* 3. Decreased pH and pO_2 and increased pCO_2.
4. Decreased pH, pCO_2, and pO_2.

Although the next question employs a different approach from the previous examples. it, too, is concerned with OXYGEN.

X. Miss Dawson is employing pursed-lip breathing. The rationale for the use of this breathing technique is to

1. increase the patency of the bronchial tree on expiration.
* 2. increase the retention of oxygen to the alveolar sacs.
3. decrease the amount of secretions in the tracheobronchial tree.
4. decrease the apprehension due to the shortness of breath.

ORGANIZING AN EXAMINATION

After all of the test questions have been written and/or retrieved from the item reservoir, the test needs to be organized before it is typed. Why should you not just turn all of the questions over to a secretary for final typing? The reasons for organizing a test involve several matters. First of all, consideration must be given to whether the items should be organized by type of question or by the content covered. Each of these points has advantages. It is hard for students to shift gears from one item format to another repeatedly. For example, to have several multiple-choice items and then to come upon a true/false question with no directions or instructions is rather startling. Since one of the maxims of test administration involves making the testing situation as free from disturbing elements as possible so that students can focus on the content aspect, this practice would violate that maxim. The other matter of organizing by content has the advantage for the student of being able to deal with everything he or she knows about cystic fibrosis or myocardial infarction or whatever. Again the student doesn't have to switch gears. To come upon a question on cancer in adults, followed by one on diabetes mellitus in children, followed by one on infectious hepatitis would be a little unnerving for the best of students. A word of caution against labeling the section with the content that is being tested. If, for example, a section of the test deals with heart conditions, a question that appears later may have heart conditions as the correct answer. The same matter applies to linking a test question to an objective in the test. If the student knows the objective, it may offer a clue to the correct answer.

Another reason for organizing the test is to avoid providing unintended clues to the correct answer. It is not uncommon for one question to provide a clue to the correct answer to another, even with experienced test writers. Sometimes the clue appears in the situation that accompanies the question and sometimes in the stem of a question. By reading through the whole test before it is typed it may help to eliminate those unintended clues.

When it is possible to do so, try to begin with one or two easy questions. It gives the student a psychological edge in that it makes them feel the test isn't going to be too bad. Of course when you organize by case situations and present a client's history and progress logically, this matter of providing an easy question first may be precluded. However, even in the case situation format, it may be possible to begin with an easy question. Unless you have used a question before and have item statistics on that item, it may not be possible to identify the item's difficulty level. Sometimes an item you think is going to be easy turns out to be more difficult than expected.

When reading through the items, make sure that each multiple-choice question uses either letters or numbers. Change those that need changing. When a number of faculty contribute items to a test, this inconsistency may crop up. (In this situation, one faculty member should be responsible for the test--organizing, proofing, etc.) Also if standard answer sheets are used, the options will need to conform to what the format is on the answer sheets.

When combination-type multiple-choice items contain the options "All of the above" and/or "None of the above" try to keep them in the same position in each item. Such consistency allows the student to spend more time on answering the question and less time searching for the answer.

When you have read through the whole test and are satisfied that it is the best that it can be, take a look at only the correct answers to see if there is a pattern of responses. When I write test questions, I very often will make my correct answer #3 unless it involves number options where they will be logically presented. If there are too many #1 and not enough #4, change those where logic is not involved. Do not, however, change those that should be presented from low to high or vice versa or where consistency is involved such as in the combination-type items. If you have 100 multiple-choice items with 4 options, about 25% of the time option number one should be correct, option two correct 25% of the time etc. With combination-type multiple-choice items when "All of the above" and/or "None of the above" are offered , they should not always be correct. About 25% of the time "All of the above" should be correct and about 25% of the time "None of the above" should be correct. The student very often will be able to deduce a particular faculty member's penchant for always having "All of the above" correct when it is offered as a choice. (Of course with computers, not only can you change at random the position of options but questions as well. The questions, however, should not be taken out of a client situation but should be independent ones.)

Now that the test is ready to be typed, some consideration should be given to how the finished test should look. Appearance is important but more important is ease of reading and responding to the questions. I can not emphasize enough that adequate spacing will facilitate test-taking. Questions and options should not be squeezed together so that options cannot be differentiated from either the stem or the next set of options. Each option should be on a separate line, not spread out across the page. Space between questions as well as between options is important. One important point that needs to be communicated to the secretary is that all parts of a question must appear on the same page. The exception to this rule involves large diagrams or pictorial material that must be presented on a separate page. In this latter situation, the graphic material should preferably be on a facing page. It is frustrating to students to have to flip through several pages to find what they need. If there is a great deal of such material that must accompany a test, it may be wise to have it presented in a separate packet. It may be helpful to present a secretary (especially a new one) with a sample page. Another thought that comes to mind is the need to caution secretaries about leaving secure materials such as tests on their desks for all to see. Tests that are in the process of being typed should be treated as strictly confidential material! In addition, they should be reminded of destroying material pertaining to the test in such a manner that it cannot be reconstructed. Papers should be shredded or torn before discarding them. When the secretary has finished typing the test, all materials should be hand-carried to you and not placed on your desk or in your open mail box.

Now that you are ready to proofread the test, several points need to be made. First, make sure that all parts of a question are there and that pieces or parts have not inadvertantly been left out. In addition to checking for typos, make sure that the test is easy to read and that all parts pertaining to an option are there. It is also important to make sure that there aren't two of question number 5 or two options number 3.

Last but not least, make sure that appropriate information is typed at the top such as the name of the school or college, space for the student to write their name, the course name and number and like and there should be complete and appropriate directions for the student.

General information that should be included in the directions for each type of item include;

1. How the student is to record the answers and where.
2. The basis upon which to select his or her answers.
3. The scoring procedure that will be used including whether or not a correction for guessing formula will be used. (It is generally not advocated to use this formula in traditional teacher-made tests.)
4. The time parameters. (In the health professions we are more likely to administer power tests

rather than speeded ones. All students should have adequate time to attempt to answer the majority of questions. Of course there are students who will sit there until next Christmas if you'll let them!)

Specific samples of directions have been included along with the examples of each type of question. See those models for further clarification.

One approach to the organization of test questions discussed earlier dealt with organizing by content. The next examples illustrate how two different types of questions that assess maternity nursing knowledge can be presented.

<u>SAMPLE OF TWO TYPES OF QUESTIONS USED WITH ONE PATIENT SITUATION</u>

(MATERNITY NURSING)

1. A woman in labor exhibits the following electronic FHR tracing:

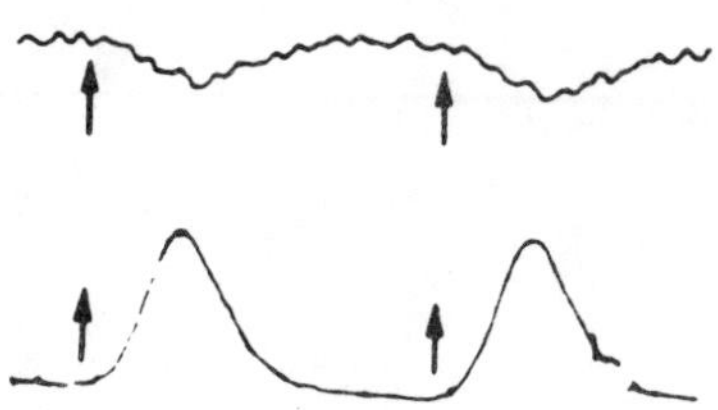

What type of deceleration pattern does this tracing demonstrate? ____(Early)____

2. The most appropriate nursing intervention for this woman would be to

    1. adjust the maternal position.
  * 2. continue to observe the patient.
    3. correct the maternal hypotension.
    4. enhance the maternal-fetal oxygen gradient.

SAMPLE OF TWO TYPES OF QUESTIONS USED WITH ONE PATIENT SITUATION

(MATERNITY NURSING)

1. A woman in labor exhibits the following electronic FHR tracing:

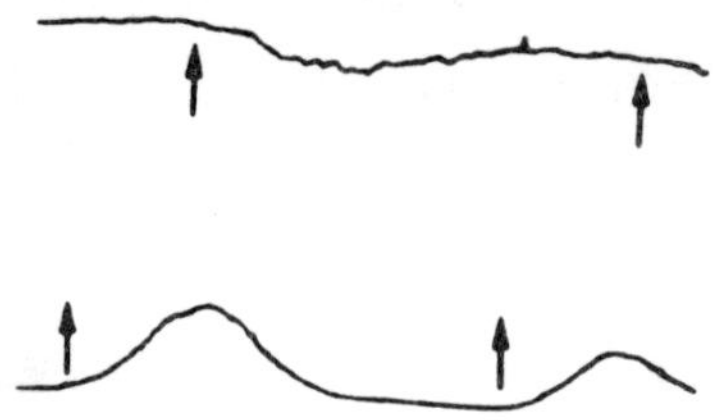

What type of deceleration pattern does this tracing demonstrate? (Late with the absence of a base line)

2. Which of the following nursing interventions would be appropriate for this woman?

   A. Elevate the vertex
   B. Administer oxygen
   C. Avoid the supine position
   D. Stop any oxytocin infusion

   1. A and C
   2. B and D
   * 3. B, C, and D
   4. All of them

TEST FORMATS

In deciding how to have your test typed, you may wish to give consideration to several popular layouts. You are probably all familiar with both of the common ones--multiple-choice items that run across the page and a two-column format such as one sees in daily newspapers, text books, and magazines. There are others that may involve a combination of those mentioned and may be dependent on whether pictorial material such as graphs or charts are a part of the testing material.

My personal preference is for the two-column format because I believe the material can be read faster. The major disadvantage I see with the two-column format is that long questions may require one side of a page. Even though this may seem like a waste of space, I think the method is justifiable based on the fact that reading is facilitated.

Other factors that may enter into any decisions about format pertain to the skill of the typist and probably to some extent, the kind of equipment on hand. Undoubtedly word processors will have a major impact on test format in the near future.

Regardless of the format chosen, I strongly recommend that material be reproduced with quality equipment so copies are legible (although I love purple, ditto copies are hard to read, especially when they have been used over and over again). Copy should not be reduced in size because readability will be affected. Graphs, charts, and pictures, however, may be reduced if their size warrants reduction. Be sure, though, that the material once reduced is legible.

A sample page of the two-column test format follows.

SAMPLE PAGE OF TWO-COLUMN TEST FORMAT

The next section of the test consists of individual items.

1. Which dietary element should be stressed by the nurse in counseling an elderly client in the maintenance of normal bowel function?
   1. Fats.
   * 2. Fiber.
   3. Minerals.
   4. Carbohydrates.

2. Which of these foods should be stressed by the nurse in counseling an elderly client in the maintenance of normal body function ?
   1. Fish.
   2. White bread.
   * 3. Fresh fruit.
   4. Mashed potatoes.

3. A nurse goes out to her car and sees her neighbor lying face down in his yard. What should the nurse do first ?
   1. Scream for help.
   2. Check his pupils.
   3. Attempt to arouse him.
   * 4. Establish an open airway.

4. The physician orders atropine gr 1/300. The atropine solution on hand contains 0.4 mg/cc. How much of the solution should be given?
   * 1. 0.5 cc
   2. 0.25 cc
   3. 1.0 cc
   4. 1.25 cc

5. Mrs. Bell, a 21-year-old primigravida, tells the nurse in the Emergency Room that she has been bleeding for the last 2 hours. In addition to assessing the nature of the bleeding, the nurse carries out three of the following actions. Which one is INAPPROPRIATE ?
   1. Evaluate the client's pain.
   2. Determine the number of weeks of gestation.
   3. Assess the client's level of apprehension.
   * 4. Assess the amount of dilatation and effacement.

6. In planning for the postpartum teaching of a primipara who delivered 2 days ago, what should be the goal of the nurse's initial encounter with the mother ?
   * 1. To determine what the mother already knows about her care.
   2. To determine the financial status of the mother.
   3. To ascertain the intellectual capacity of the mother.
   4. To ascertain the support systems available to the mother following her discharge.

GO ON TO THE NEXT PAGE

SECTION 4: ITEM ANALYSIS

DEFINITIONS AND OBTAINING THE UPPER AND LOWER GROUPS FOR ITEM ANALYSIS

Difficulty level or index -- the percentage of the group that answered the item correctly. If 70 percent of the examinees answered the item correctly, the item has a 70 percent difficulty.

Discrimination index or power -- the ability of an item to differentiate the high-scoring group from the low-scoring group. Ideally, the brighter students answer the item correctly while the less able students do not.

Obtaining the upper and lower groups for the purpose of item analysis

After the test has been scored, the papers should be arranged from the highest scorer to the lowest scorer. Then divide the papers into three piles--the top 25 percent, the middle 50 percent, and the lowest 25 percent. The top 25 percent becomes the upper group and the lowest 25 percent becomes the lower group. For most ordinary classroom situations, it is not necessary to deal with the middle group because the data derived from its inclusion differs very little from those obtained using the upper and lower groups.

The next step is to total all of the answers chosen for each item for each group. For example, for item #1, suppose that 18 students in the upper group answered the item correctly but only 6 students in the lower group answered the item correctly. It can then be said that the item is discriminating positively and in the desired direction.

An item analysis card on page 176 illustrates the recording of the numbers of students in each of the two groups who answered an item correctly. An alternate format is shown on page 179.

ITEM ANALYSIS

Test questions cannot be written at a specified level of difficulty. What may seem to be a difficult concept may turn out to be relatively easy and vice versa. It is not possible to determine either whether distractors will work or not, even though we attempt to write only plausible options. Item analysis enters the picture at this point (following test administration, of course), and provides answers by way of the data generated.

Item analysis data provide information about:

1. Which distractors did not work and which one(s) worked best;
2. Whether an item was hard or easy;
3. Did the item effectively discriminate the better students from the less able ones.

In addition, item analysis data may also point to problems in the item such as ambiguity and the possibility of an unintended second or alternate best answer.

If distractors do not function as intended, if no one chose it or a very small number chose it, the distractor(s) should be revised before the item is used again. If, however, an item is very easy, say 98% difficulty (think easiness), it should be obvious that one or more distractors are not working. Since only a small sample of the universe of content of a given subject is usually tested, I believe that all items should be important ones and functional, contributing to the assessment process. An item that is so easy that most examinees get it correct, is not serving much of a function. There are instances, however, when you will want to administer questions that assess essential content when it is hoped that most students will answer correctly. Items pertaining to sterile technique, CPR, patient safety, and the like fall into this mastery category.

There is also a relationship between the difficulty of an item and the discrimination power of that item. If the item is very easy, 98% or 100% of the students answering correctly, the discrimination power will be around .00. An item that 50% of the students get correct--all of them in the upper group answering correctly and none of them in the lower group getting it correct--the discrimination power will be 1.00, or the maximum discrimination power possible. For this reason, faculty are encouraged to write and use items at the 50% level of difficulty.

Although there are rather simple methods for calculating item difficulty and discrimination power (using either upper and lower groups of 25% or 27%), the availability of computers has provided many faculty with item analysis printouts based on the total group. A word of caution, though, regarding the interpretation of item statistics based on small groups. Indices of difficulty and discrimination power are likely to vary from group to group so that an accumulation of such data from several small groups (and recorded on the item card) will be more reliable.

My purpose for including this section is not to teach you everything you need to know about item analysis but rather to show you how to use the data in order to improve the statistical properties or characteristics of the items and the item itself. First the item in its original form will be presented, then the item analysis data for that item, followed by my comments regarding the data as applied to that item, and in some instances, a revision of the item based on the data.

The fifteen items along with their item analysis were contributed by Dr. June Lawrence, Associate Professor in the School of Nursing of the University of Mississippi at the Medical Center. I am most appreciative of her interest in the book and her willingness to share her products.

ITEM ANALYSIS CARD (1)

Course: Dates used:

Content: Key:

Objective:

Item

What is the generic name for the drug Miltown?

A. Darvon.

B. Equinal.

* C. Meprobamate.

D. Salicylic Acid.

Student Responses:

Percent	Alternative	Upper	Lower	Total
	A.			
	B.			
	C.			
	D.			

Item Difficulty __________ Discrimination Power__________

Recommendations:

ITEM ANALYSIS CARD (2)

Course: Maternal-Newborn Nursing N-325 Item Number: 17

Objective: Uses the appropriate sequence of steps in assessing fetal heart tones.

Key: 4

Item: Which of these actions should most certainly have been taken by the nurse prior to listening to the fetal heart rate?

1. Counting the mother's radial pulse.
2. Ascertaining the height of the uterine fundus.
3. Determining the station of the fetus.
4. Palpating the abdomen for fetal position.

Options	1	2	3	4	5	Omits
Upper 25% (12 students)	0	0	0	12	0	0
Lower 25% (12 students)	2	3	2	5	0	0

Difficulty = 71%

Discrimination = .58

ITEM ANALYSIS CARD (3)

FRONT OF CARD

Course: Client as a System III

Objective: Identify the incidence of common urinary tract infections in children.

Item: Which of the following statements about the incidence of urinary tract infections in children is true?

A. It is a low incidence problem that is easily cleared by treatment with medication, even though recurrence is a possibility.

B. It is a high incidence problem but usually is nonrecurring.

* C. It is a high incidence problem because it is both common in many children and tends to recur.

D. It is high incidence problem that has even surpassed the incidence or respiratory infections.

BACK OF CARD

Date	9/17/82			
Number in Class	75			
Percentage Correct	51%			
Correct Answer	C			
Option A	35 47%			
B	2 3%			
C	38 51%			
D	0 0			
Discrimination Index	+.30			
R Point Biserial	+.19			

COMMENTS: Revise D. It is a high incidence problem and is equivalent in incidence to that of respiratory infections.

ITEM ANALYSIS CARD (4)

FRONT OF CARD

Course: Client as a System III

Objective: Identify the incidence of common urinary tract infections in children.

Item: Which of the following statements about the incidence of urinary tract infections in children is true?

A. It is a low incidence problem that is easily cleared by treatment with medication, even though recurrence is a possibility.

B. It is a high incidence problem but usually is nonrecurring.

* C. It is a high incidence problem because it is both common in many children and tends to recur.

D. It is a high incidence problem that has even surpassed the incidence or respiratory infections.

TEST DATE	Dec. '82	April '83	Dec. '83		
ITEM NO.	15	22	13		

REVERSE SIDE OF CARD

ITEM RECORD												
UPPER						LOWER						
DATE	A	B	C	D	Omits	A	B	C	D	Omits	% Correct	Dis.
Dec. '82												
April '83												
Dec. '83												

ORIGINAL QUESTION

1. The number of repeated urine cultures for bacteria colony count can be reduced by the nurse's careful cleansing of the perineum and collection of a midstream specimen and by testing the urine prior to sending it to the lab for

* A. specific gravity.
B. presence of protein.
C. presence of glucose.
D. presence of ketones.

Date	9/17/82		
Number in class	75		
Percentage correct	40%		
Correct answer	A		
Option A	30 40%		
B	23 31%		
C	16 21%		
D	6 8%		
Discrimination Index	+.30		
R Point Biserial	+.19		

NOTE: The discrimination index reported in the item analysis is based on the upper 27% of the 75 students and the lower 27% of the 75 students. The R Point Biserial reported here is based on the total group of 75 students.

I have used the discrimination index in my comments rather than the R Point Biserial, reported automatically in our item analysis statistics at the Medical Center. Therefore, you may wish to consult any of the following texts, as well as others currently available, for information on the R Point Biserial.

Guilford, J. P. and B. Fruchter. 1977. Fundamental Statistics in Psychology and Education. 6th ed. McGraw-Hill Book Co., New York.

Hopkins, K. D. and J. C. Stanley. 1981. Educational and Psychological Measurement and Evaluation. 6th ed. Prentice-Hall, Inc., Englewood Cliffs, New Jersey.

Kurtz, A. K. and S. T. Mayo. 1979. Statistical Methods in Education and Psychology. Springer-Verlag, New York.

COMMENTS

The item is rather difficult even though the correct answer is different from the other options. Each of the distractors is working. The discrimination index is good. The data does not warrant changing the item but because of test construction reasons I would make the following changes.

Because the stem is long and difficult to understand, I would make it two sentences. I also wonder if the first part of the stem is necessary. You could start the item with "Prior to sending a urine specimen to the lab for culture, the nurse should test the urine for" which would become your new stem. I would try to change at least one of the distractors, B, C, or D to make it parallel with the correct answer, A.

ORIGINAL QUESTION

2. A voiding cystograph is used to detect

A. hypospadius.
B. urinary retention due to ureteropelvic stenosis.
* C. urinary retention due to vesicoureteral reflux.
D. abnormal force and volume of the urine flow during voiding.

Date	9/17/82		
Number in class	75		
Percentage correct	93%		
Correct answer	C		
Option A	2 3%		
B	1 1%		
C	70 93%		
D	2 3%		
Discrimination Index	+.05		
R Point Biserial	+.06		

COMMENTS

It is an easy item--93% got it correct. The low discrimination index is related to the easiness of the item. Was this item near item number 3 originally? The correct answer contains the words vesicoureteral reflux which is the stem of the next question. Change option B because only 1 person chose it. It may make the item a little harder.

REVISED QUESTION

2. A voiding cystograph is used to detect

A. hypospadius.
B. ureteropelvic stenosis.
* C. urinary retention due to vesicoureteral reflux.
D. abnormal force and volume of the urine flow during voiding.

NOTE: Any time that a distractor is revised, it should be validated to make sure that it is incorrect.

ORIGINAL QUESTION

3. Recurrent urinary tract infection (UTI) may be associated with vesicoureteral reflux, which is

A. congenital malformation involving the kidney pelvis with its junction or formation into the ureter producing stenosis and retention.
B. a malformation of the urethra near the bladder producing retention and resulting bladder distention.
* C. a malfunction of the flap-like valve formed by the oblique passage of the ureter through the bladder muscle and mucous membrane lining.
D. a neurogenically damaged bladder.

Date	9/17/82			
Number in class	75			
Percentage correct	96%			
Correct answer	C			
Option A	1	1%		
B	2	3%		
C	72	96%		
D	0	0		
Discrimination Index	+.10			
R Point Biserial	+.16			

COMMEMTS

It is an easy item since 96% got it right. The discrimination index is low in part because the item is very easy. Since no one chose option D, change it significantly. By changing D, more people might choose A and B, as well as D. Since the correct answer sounds so specific, I wonder if it was taken directly from the text. It would be better to revise the correct answer using your own words.

From a test construction point of view, the first part of the stem is a teaching phrase. Begin the stem of the question with "The definition of vesicoureteral reflux is."

ORIGINAL VERSION

4. Successful treatment of urinary tract infection (UTI) may be dependent upon which of the following in addition to appropriate antimicrobial therapy?

   A. Maintaining adequate milk and protein intake.
   B. Prevention of vigorous physical activity.
   C. Reduction of salty foods such as potato chips in the diet.
 * D. Prevention of constipation.

Date	9/17/82			
Number in class	75			
Percentage correct	48%			
Correct answer	D			
Option A	8	11%		
B	13	17%		
C	18	24%		
D	36	48%		
Discrimination Index	+.10			
R Point Biserial	+.11			

COMMENTS

The difficulty level is appropriate since approximately 50% got it right. Each of the distractors is working. The discrimination index is low, however, so it would be wise to edit the item and try it again. If after editing the item and trying it out again and the data remains essentially unchanged, then perhaps more stringent revisions will need to be made.

REVISED QUESTION

4. In addition to appropriate antimicrobial therapy, successful treatment of urinary tract infection (UTI) may be dependent upon which of the following measures?

   A. Maintenance of an adequate milk and protein intake.
   B. Prevention of vigorous physical activity.
   C. Reduction of salty foods in the diet such as potato chips.
   * D. Prevention of constipation.

ORIGINAL QUESTION

5. Urinary tract infection (UTI) recurrence should be evaluated with a thorough physical examination and tests of normality of renal structure and function because

   A. this is most likely associated with already existing renal function damage.
   * B. there may be congenital malformations that will need surgical intervention.
   C. this is a painful and emotionally traumatic problem.
   D. this may be a chronic illness that needs psychological intervention to determine if masturbation may be a contributing factor.

Date	9/17/82		
Number in class	75		
Percentage correct	87%		
Correct answer	B		
Option A	9 12%		
B	65 87%		
C	0 0		
D	1 1%		
Discrimination Index	+.20		
R Point Biserial	+.19		

COMMENTS

The item is a relatively easy one since 87% of the students answered correctly. No one chose option C and only one student chose option D. The discrimination index is satisfactory. By revising (editing) the stem and the options, the data may change for the better. The stem of the question should be closed in this question to make it easier to read and answer.

REVISED QUESTION

5. The recurrence of urinary tract infections (UTI) should be evaluated with a thorough physical examination and tests of normality of renal structure and function for which of these reasons?

   A. Renal function damage may already be present and can be treated.
 * B. Congenital malformations may be present that will need surgical intervention.
   C. Psychological intervention may be indicated to determine if masturbation may be a contributing factor.
   D. Pain and emotional trauma associated with the condition will be minimized.

ORIGINAL QUESTION

6. The nurse is assigned to a male preschooler, who is to have surgical repair for hypospadius. The nurse should consider a normal or common concern of boys at this age, which is

   A. anxiety of having a "small" penis.
 * B. fear of mutilation or loss of his penis.
   C. anxiety associated with occasional eneuresis.
   D. fear of never being a "daddy."

Date	9/17/82			
Number in class	75			
Percentage correct	96%			
Correct answer	B			
Option A	1	1%		
B	72	96%		
C	0	0		
D	2	3%		
Discrimination Index	.00			
R Point Biserial	+.03			

COMMENTS

This was a very easy item--96% choosing the correct answer. The discrimination index is .00 which indicates, of course, that there is none. Since the large majority of the students chose the correct answer, it should come as no surprise that the discrimination is .00. One way to make the item harder is to change option C since no one picked it. It would be wise to revise options A and D since only a total of 3 examinees chose those.

REVISED QUESTION

6. A male preschooler is to have a surgical repair for hypospadius. A normal or common concern of boys at this age which should be taken into consideration by the nurse is

   A. fear of never being a daddy.
 * B. fear of mutilation or loss of his penis.
   C. anxiety about having a small or different penis.
   D. anxiety about being different from others.

ORIGINAL QUESTION

7. Nephrosis is another common childhood renal problem. The most common pathophysiologic process is

A. proteinuria due to hypertension.
B. proteinuria due to increased plasma protein of unknown etiology.
* C. proteinuria due to changes in the basement membrane of the glomeruli of unknown etiology.
D. renal failure due to massive loss of fluid into the interstitial spaces.

Date	9/17/82		
Number in class	75		
Percentage correct	65%		
Correct answer	C		
Option A	5 7%		
B	16 21%		
C	49 65%		
D	5 7%		
Discrimination Index	+.25		
R Point Biserial	+.26		

COMMENTS

This item has desirable statistical properties. The difficulty level is 65%, all of the options are working, and the discrimination index is satisfactory at +.25. The only change I would make is in the stem of the question. The first sentence is unnecessary. The revised stem could read--The most common pathophysiologic process in nephrosis is, with the options as originally presented.

ORIGINAL QUESTION

8. The edema of idiopathic childhood nephrosis is

A. massive, but it responds readily to diuretic medications, such as hydrodiuril or lasix.
* B. massive, but it responds to corticosteroid therapy.
C. minimal, and it responds to antihypertensive medications, such as apresoline.
D. minimal, and it responds to bedrest and reduced fluid intake.

Date	9/17/82			
Number in class	75			
Percentage correct	51%			
Correct answer	B			
Option A	10	13%		
B	38	51%		
C	14	19%		
D	13	17%		
Discrimination Index	+.50			
R Point Biserial	+.37			

COMMENTS

This item has outstanding item characteristics. The difficulty level is 51%, all of the distractors are working about equally, and the discrimination index is great at +.50. I would make no changes except in option A. I would change the or to and.

ORIGINAL QUESTION

Tim Avery, a previously healthy 8-year-old boy, has been admitted to the hospital with a tentative diagnosis of acute glomerulonephritis.

9. Acute glomerulonephritis (AGN) is

A. an infection of the glomeruli of the kidney.
B. an infection of the glomeruli of the kidney with streptococci found in the urine culture.
* C. an immune complex reaction.
D. a frequent initial cause of chronic renal failure in children.

Date	9/17/82			
Number in class	75			
Percentage correct	48%			
Correct answer	C			
Option A	20	27%		
B	14	19%		
C	36	48%		
D	5	7%		
Discrimination Index	+.70			
R Point Biserial	+.52			

COMMENTS

The difficulty level of this item is slightly on the hard side at 48% and all of the distractors are working. The discrimination index is outstanding at +.70! In spite of these outstanding characteristics, I suggest revising the stem in order to let the examinees know what they are supposed to look for--in this instance a description. Because the stem is to be revised, the options will also need to be changed to go with the stem. I would also delete the word culture in option B.

REVISED QUESTION

9. Which of these descriptions is accurate about acute glomerulonephritis (AGN)?

   A. It is an infection of the glomeruli of the kidney.
   B. It is an infection of the glomeruli of the kidney with streptococci found in the urine.
   * C. It is an immune complex reaction.
   D. It is a frequent initial cause of chronic renal failure in children.

ORIGINAL QUESTION

10. The initial assessment of the nurse should include collection of a urine specimen to

* A. observe the color.
B. determine specific gravity, which will be decreased.
C. obtain an immediate "dipstick" reading for proteinuria and glucosuria.
D. send a specimen to the laboratory for culture.

Date	9/17/82			
Number in class	75			
Percentage correct	65%			
Correct answer	A			
Option A	49	65%		
B	10	13%		
C	15	20%		
D	1	1%		
Discrimination Index	+.10			
R Point Biserial	+.10			

COMMENTS

The difficulty level of 65% is satisfactory and options B and C are working well. Since only 1 examinee chose option D, it should be revised. The discrimination index of +.10 is too low. By revising option D, it may positively affect the discrimination index. This item had been preceded by the situation given in the previous question. By relocating that situation, it may have an effect on the item analysis of this item as well as the previous one and the one that follows.

REVISED QUESTION

10. The initial assessment by the nurse should include the collection of a urine specimen from Tim in order to

   * A. observe the color.
   B. determine the specific gravity, which will be decreased.
   C. obtain an immediate "dipstick" reading for proteinuria and glucosuria.
   D. send a specimen to the laboratory for culture and sensitivity studies.

ORIGINAL QUESTION

11. On day three (3) of his admission, Tim's condition worsens. During your early assessment, you find that Tim's blood pressure is elevated to 146/92. He has not voided since 8:00 p.m. and his bladder is not distended. Considering possible complications, which of the following nursing actions would be most appropriate initially?

    A. Notify the physician of your observation of hypertension when the physician makes his daily rounds.
  * B. Maintain bedrest and assess for unusual neurologic symptoms, such as headache, blurred vision, irritability or vomiting.
    C. Have Tim drink several glasses of water to determine if his lack of voiding is due to inadequate intake.
    D. Immediately notify the physician of his hypertension.

Date	9/17/82			
Number in class	75			
Percentage correct	55%			
Correct answer	B			
Option A	4	5%		
B	41	55%		
C	1	1%		
D	29	39%		
Discrimination Index	+.25			
R Point Biserial	+.17			

COMMENTS

The difficulty level of 55% is quite appropriate and the discrimination index of +.25 is satisfactory. Option D worked very effectively but only 1 person chose option C and only 4 examinees chose option A. I would therefore change options A and C. The correct answer contains more than one part. I would, therefore, add additional parts to other options. See the revised options A and C.

REVISED QUESTION

11. On the third day after his admission, Tim's condition worsens. During his early assessment, Tim's blood pressure is elevated to 146/92. He has not voided since 8:00 p.m. but his bladder is not distended. Which of the following nursing actions would be most appropriate initially?

    A. Recheck his blood pressure in the other arm using another cuff.
    B. Immediately notify the physician of Tim's hypertension.
    C. Ask Tim if he needs to void and offer him a urinal.
    * D. Maintain bedrest and assess him for unusual neurologic symptoms, such as headache, blurred vision, irritability, and vomiting.

ORIGINAL QUESTION

12. Unwed adolescent pregnancy is most often the result of

A. an impulsive but accidental, spontaneous expression of love.
B. a lack of knowledge related to the need for, as well as the effective use of contraception.
C. a lack of available contraception services and contraceptive devices.
* D. fulfillment of a need for the girl associated with the developmental changes of adolescence.

Date	10/1/82		
Number in class	74		
Percentage correct	57 77%		
Correct answer	D		
Option A	6 8%		
B	11 15%		
C	0		
D	57 77%		
Discrimination Index	+.35		
R Point Biserial	+.20		

COMMENTS

The difficulty level of 77% is perfectly acceptable, especially since the discrimination index is +.35. The only real problem with this item, in terms of the item analysis, is the fact that no one chose option C. Therefore, option C needs to be revised. In so doing, it may make the item a little harder which would be desirable.

From a test construction point of view, there is a clue in the stem to the correct answer. I would put the word adolescent or adolescence in options A and C.

NOTE: There are times when it is not necessary to revise options even though no one chose them. If the difficulty level and discrimination index are satisfactory, sometimes it is wise to leave the item alone!

REVISED QUESTION

12. Unwed adolescent pregnancy is most often the result of

    A. an impulsive but accidental, spontaneous expression of adolescent love.
    B. a lack of knowledge related to the need for, as well as the effective use of contraceptives.
    C. contraception services and/or devices geared to the adolescent.
    * D. fulfillment of a need for the girl associated with the developmental changes of adolescence.

ORIGINAL QUESTION

13. The incidence of adolescent pregnancy is

A. reflecting an overall increasing fertility rate in the United States.
B. increasing, but the percentage of births to adolescents as compared with total births is decreasing.
* C. resulting in 20% of all children in the United States being born to adolescents.
D. resulting in a current increase in adolescent marriages.

Date	10/1/82		
Number in class	74		
Percentage correct	64 86%		
Correct answer	C		
Option A	0		
B	8 11%		
C	64 86%		
D	2 3%		
Discrimination Index	+.00		
R Point Biserial	+.03		

COMMENTS

The item is quite easy with a difficulty level of 86%. The item does not discriminate at all since the index is .00. No one chose option A so it will need to be changed. I would revise the item and try it again.

REVISED QUESTION

13. The incidence of adolescent pregnancy in the United States is

A. reflected in an overall increased fertility rate.
B. producing an increase currently in adolescent marriages.
* C. resulting in 20% of all children being born to adolescents.
D. increasing, but the percentage of births to adolescents as compared with total births is decreasing.

ORIGINAL QUESTION

14. The two (2) most common physical health problems of pregnant adolescents are iron deficiency anemia and

A. prolonged nausea and vomiting.
B. hypoglycemia in the early morning hours.
* C. preeclampsia.
D. gestational diabetes.

Date	10/1/82		
Number in class	74		
Percentage correct	73 99%		
Correct answer	C		
Option A	0		
B	0		
C	73 99%		
D (1 student chose E)	0		
Discrimination Index	+.00		
R Point Biserial	-.01		

COMMENTS

All but one student answered this item correctly--the difficulty level is 99%. One student answered E but since there was no option E, it was probably an error in recording the answer on the answer sheet. It should not be surprising that there is no discrimination index in light of the easiness of the item. I would revise the item and try it again.

REVISED QUESTION

14. In addition to iron deficiency anemia, the most common health problem of pregnant adolescents is

A. malnutrition.
B. hypoglycemia.
*C. preeclampsia,
D. severe nausea and vomiting.

ORIGINAL QUESTION

15. The most typical description of the father of the baby of an unwed adolescent is that

* A. he is a member of her peer group and that he wants to share in the decisions and responsibilities associated with the pregnancy.
  B. he is a member of her peer group but that he takes no responsibility associated with the pregnancy because he has already impregnanted several girls.
  C. he is an adolescent several years older than the girl and that he has initiated an unwilling girl into sexual activity.
  D. he is an adult man who has taken advantage of the girl's youth and lack of heterosexual experience.

Date	10/1/82		
Number in class	74		
Percentage correct	97%		
Correct answer	A		
Option A	72 97%		
B	2 3%		
C	0		
D	0		
Discrimination Index	+.05		
R Point Biserial	+.13		

COMMENTS

The item is very easy in that all of the students answered correctly except for 2 of them. The low discrimination index of +.05 is related to the easiness of the item. Options C and D need to be changed since no one chose them which will probably affect the difficulty level, making the item harder.

REVISED QUESTION

15. Which of the following descriptions is most typical of the father of the baby of an unwed adolescent?

* A. He is a member of her peer group and wants to share in the decisions and responsibilities associated with the pregnancy.
  B. He is a member of her peer group but takes no responsibility associated with the pregnancy because he probably has already impregnated several other girls.
  C. He is an adult who is willing to support the baby but assume no other responsibilities in relation to child rearing.
  D. He is an adolescent who at times manifests adult behavior except when it pertains to his girlfriend and the unwanted pregnancy.

REFERENCES

BOOKS:

Adkins, D.C. 1974. Test Construction. 2nd ed. Charles E. Merrill Co., Columbus, Ohio.

Ahmann, J.S. and M.D. Glock. 1981. Evaluating Student Progress. 6th ed. Allyn and Bacon, Inc., Boston.

Anastasi, A. 1982. Psychological Testing. 5th ed. Macmillan Publishing Co., Inc., New York.

Berk, R.A. (Ed.). 1980. Criterion-Referenced Measurement. The State of the Art. The Johns Hopkins University Press, Baltimore.

Bloom, B.S.; T.J. Hastings; and G. Madaus. 1971. Handbook on Formative and Summative Evaluation of Student Learning. McGraw-Hill Book Co., New York.

Bloom, B.S.; G. Madaus; and T.J. Hastings. 1980. Evaluation to Improve Learning. McGraw-Hill Book Co., New York.

Bormuth, J.R. 1970. On the Theory of Achievement Test Items. The University of Chicago Press, Chicago.

Brightwell, D.S. and M.L. Howard. 1976. Individualized Learning Modules for Norman E. Gronlund's Measurement and Evaluation in Teaching. 3rd. ed. Macmillan Publishing Co., Inc., New York.

Brown, F.G. 1980. Guidelines for Test Use: A Commentary on the Standards for Educational and Psychological Tests. National Council on Measurement in Education.

Capobianco, A.T. 1979. The Development of a System for Evaluation. National League for Nursing, New York.

Cronbach, L.J. 1970. Essentials of Psychological Testing. 3rd. ed. Harper and Row, Publishers, New York.

Dvorak, E.M. and others. 1982. The National Council Licensure Examination for Registered Nurses. Chicago Review Press, Chicago.

Ebel, R.L. 1979. Essentials of Educational Measurement. 3rd ed. Prentice-Hall, Inc., Englewood Cliffs, N.J.

Frisbie, D.A. 1979. Evaluating Student Achievement: Principles, Trends, and Problems. National League for Nursing, New York.

Gronlund, N.E. 1982. Constructing Achievement Tests. 3rd ed. Prentice-Hall., Englewood Cliffs, N.J.

Gronlund, N.E. 1981. Measurement and Evaluation in Teaching. 4th ed. Macmillan Publishing Co., New York.

Gronlund, N.E. 1973. Preparing Criterion-Referenced Tests for Classroom Instruction. Macmillan Publishing Co., New York.

Gronlund, N.E. 1978. Stating Objectives for Classroom Instruction. 2nd ed. Macmillan Publishing Co., New York.

Guilford, J.P. and B. Fruchter. 1977. Fundamental Statistics in Psychology and Education. 6th ed. McGraw-Hill Book Co., New York.

Hopkins, C.D. and R.L. Antes. 1978. Classroom Measurement and Evaluation. F.E. Peacock Publishers, Inc., Itasca, Illinois.

Hopkins, K.D. and J.C. Stanley. 1981. Educational and Psychological Measurement and Evaluation. 6th ed. Prentice-Hall, Inc., Englewood Cliffs, N.J.

Hubbard, J.P. 1978. Measuring Medical Education. The Tests and Experience of the National Board of Medical Examiners. 2nd ed. Lea and Febiger, Philadelphia.

King, E.C. 1979. Classroom Evaluation Strategies. C.V. Mosby Co., St. Louis.

Lyman, H.B. 1978. Test Scores and What They Mean. 3rd ed. Prentice-Hall, Inc., Englewood Cliffs, N.J.

Magnusson, D. 1967. Test Theory. Addison-Wesley Publishing Co., Reading, Mass.

Mehrens, W.A. and I.J. Lehmann. 1978. Measurement and Evaluation in Education and Psychology. 2nd ed. Holt, Rinehart and Winston, Inc., New York.

Morris, L.L. and C.T. Fitz-Gibbon. 1978. How to Measure Achievement. Sage Publications, Beverly Hills, Calif.

National League for Nursing. 1979. Developing Tests to Evaluate Student Achievement in Baccalaureate Nursing Programs. Pub. No. 15-1761. National League for Nursing, New York.

National League for Nursing. 1965. Pamphlet No. 5: The Construction and Use of Teacher Made Tests. National League for Nursing, New York.

Nunnally, J.C. 1978. Psychometric Theory. McGraw-Hill Book Co., New York.

Payne, D.A. 1974. The Assessment of Learning: Cognitive and Affective. D.C. Heath and Company, Lexington, Mass.

Payne, D.A. (Ed.). 1974. Curriculum Evaluation: Commentaries on Purpose, Process and Product. D.C. Heath and Company, Lexington, Mass.

Payne, D.A. and R.F. McMorris. 1975. Educational and Psychological Measurement. 2nd ed. General Learning Press, Morristown, N.J.

Popham, W.J. (Ed.). 1971. Criterion-Referenced Measurement. (An Introduction). Educational Technology Publications, Englewood Cliffs, N.J.

Popham, W.J. 1978. Criterion-Referenced Measurement. Prentice-Hall, Inc., Englewood Cliffs, N.J.

Popham, W.J. 1975. Educational Evaluation. Prentice-Hall, Inc., Englewood Cliffs, N.J.

Popham, W.J. (Ed.). 1974. Evaluation in Education: Current Applications. McCutchan Publishing Corp., Berkeley, Calif.

Popham, W.J. and E.L. Baker. 1970. Systematic Instruction. Prentice-Hall, Inc., Englewood Cliffs, N.J.

Reilly, D.E. 1980. Behavioral Objectives--Evaluation in Nursing. 2nd ed. Appleton-Century-Crofts, New York.

Rezler, A.G. and B.J. Stevens. (Eds.). 1978. The Nurse Evaluator in Education and Service. McGraw-Hill Book Co., New York.

Roid, G.H. and T.M. Haladyna. 1982. A Technology for Test-Item Writing. Academic Press, New York.

Scannell, D.P. and D.B. Tracy. 1975. Testing and Measurement in the Classroom. Houghton Mifflin Co., Boston.

Schneider, H.L. 1979. Evaluation of Nursing Competence. H. and B. Hess Co., Jackson, MS.

Schrader, W.B. (Ed.). 1980. New Directions for Testing and Measurement--Measuring Achievement: Progress Over a Decade. Proceedings of the 1979 Educational Testing Service Invitational Conference. Jossey-Bass, Inc., San Francisco.

Testing and Public Interest. 1977. Proceedings of the 1976 Educational Testing Service Invitational Conference. Educational Testing Service, Princeton, N.J.

Thorndike, R.L. (Ed.). 1971. Educational Measurement. 2nd ed. American Council on Education, Washington, D.C.

Thorndike, R.L. and E.P. Hagen. 1977. Measurement and Evaluation in Psychology and Education. 4th ed. John Wiley and Sons, Inc., New York.

Tuckman, B.W. 1979. Evaluating Instructional Programs. Allyn and Bacon, Inc., Boston.

<u>ARTICLES</u>:

Bower, F.L. 1974. Normative -or Criterion-Referenced Evaluation? Nursing Outlook, 22(8):499-502.

Chandler, J.M. and M.L. Hunter. 1976. Teaching by Testing. Nursing Outlook, 24(6):386-388.

Ebel, R.L. 1982. Proposed Solutions to Two Problems of Test Construction. Journal of Educational Measurement, 19(4):267-278.

Frisbie, D.A. 1983. Testing Achievement Beyond the Knowledge Level. Journal of Nursing Education, 22(6): 228-231.

King, E.C. 1978. Constructing Classroom Achievement Tests. Nurse Educator, 5:30-36.

Kubo, W.; L. Chase; and J. Leton. 1971. A Creative Examination. Nursing Outlook, 19(8):524-526.

Let's Examine - Nursing Outlook. The series began in January, 1961 and appeared monthly through February, 1971. An additional six articles appeared through December, 1971.

Rezler, A.G. and R. Wang Liu. 1977. Hope for That Hopeless Essay Test. Journal of Nursing Education, 16(9):5-11.

Smith, J.K. 1982. Converging on Correct Answers: A Peculiarity of Multiple Choice Items. Journal of Educational Measurement, 19(3):211-220.

Stokes, S.A. and others. 1981. The Development of an Evaluation Process for Technical Level Competency. Nursing and Health Care, 4:192-195, 230.

Stanton, M.P.H. 1983. Objective Test Construction--A Must for Nursing Educators. Journal of Nursing Education, 22(8):338-339.

Sumida, S.W. 1972. A Computerized Test for Clinical Decision-Making. Nursing Outlook, 20(7):458-461.

Ward, J.A. and J.M. Griffin. 1977. Improving Instruction Through Computer-Graded Examinations. Nursing Outlook, 25(8):524-529.

Westwick, C.R. 1976. Item Analysis. Journal of Nursing Education, 15(5):27-32.